Your *Plus-Size* Pregnancy

Your *Plus-Size* Pregnancy

The Ultimate Guide for the Full-Figured Expectant Mom

Brette McWhorter Sember
with Bruce D. Rodgers, M.D.

**Officially Endorsed by the Department of Gynecology and Obstetrics
University at Buffalo
The State University of New York
School of Medicine and Biomedical Sciences**

BARRICADE BOOKS

Fort Lee, New Jersey

The information in this book that deals with medical, mental health, nutritional, and fitness issues is provided for basic information only. You should always consult your own health-care provider about your specific case and what is recommended for you. This book is not a substitute for medical care or advice. The authors and publisher disclaim any liability from any claims arising from any information contained in this book.

Published by Barricade Books Inc.
185 Bridge Plaza North
Suite 308-A
Fort Lee, NJ 07024

www.barricadebooks.com

Library of Congress Cataloging-in-Publication Data

Sember, Brette McWhorter, 1968-
    Your plus-size pregnancy : the ultimate guide for the full-figured expectant mom /
    Brette McWhorter Sember with Bruce D. Rogers.
        p. cm.
    Includes bibliographical references and index.
    ISBN 1-56980-290-4 (pbk.)
    1. Pregnancy--Popular works. 2. Overweight women--Health and hygiene--Popular
    works. I. Rodgers, Bruce D. II Title.

RG525.S42 2005
618.2--dc22

                                                                                    2005053017

First Printing
Printed in Canada

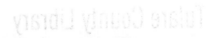

Contents

Contents

Contents

Contents

Contents

Foreword

I have been plus size for most of my 42 years and I know first-hand what it's like to live in a "skinny obsessed" world. In this world, it's a challenge to find clothes to fit. In this world, a simple checkup at the doctor's can turn into a sermon on the merits of losing weight. In this world, chairs can be too small, seat belts—too short and robes at the hairdresser's—too skimpy.

I've never been pregnant. I can only imagine how these experiences intensify for my glorious PREGNANT plus-size sisters. Living in a plus-size pregnant body cannot be for the faint of heart.

From what my friends tell me, it's a little scary to be pregnant for *any* woman. Your body changes so quickly, your emotions teeter and you are always just a tad worried for the safety and security of your unborn baby and for yourself as well. Wise words and sound information are paramount at this time and women need to know that someone else has walked in their shoes and survived it all.

Our plus-size sisters are no different than any other woman. We live, we love, we shop, we eat, we marry, we have babies. The missing link here is that we have never had the wise words or sound information that related specifically to our own fully-figured bodies. Thankfully, over the years, information has been more free-flowing in the areas of health, fashion, style, and beauty for the plus woman. But never has there been a "bible" just for us when we get pregnant.

Enter Brette Sember and the very important book you are holding in your hands right now. This book is your new best friend and primary source for every scrap of vital information you will need to have a spectacular, worry-free nine months and a safe, healthy delivery. With care, tenderness, sage words, advice from a renowned Ob-Gyn, and actual testimonials from real women, you will find answers to all the big, scary questions you have—as well as the little ones you never thought of too.

With this book, you shall go forth and multiply fearlessly with your big, beautiful body (made for childbearing, by the way) and bring into this world a delicious, healthy baby.

Courage.

—Catherine Lippincott,
Director of Public Relations and Special Events
for Charming Shoppes (Lane Bryant, Catherine's,
and Fashion Bug), plus-size model and author of
*Well Rounded: Eight Simple Steps for
Changing Your Life...Not Your Size*

Acknowledgments

This book is dedicated to the wonderful women who opened up their souls and generously shared their plus-size pregnancy experiences. I am so honored and touched by your honesty, openness, thoughtfulness, and insights.

Many thanks go to Patricia Lindsey-Salvo, Merry McVey-Noble, Lisa Stone, Merry Rose, Catherine Schuller, Rochelle Rice, Jane Hanrahan, Andrea Henderson, Ann Leach, Leanne Ely, Misty Bott, Sheri Wallace, Bonnie Bernell, Catherine Lippincott, Barbara Brickner, Wendy Shanker, Kelly Bliss, and every other professional who took the time to be interviewed for this book or to read it and discuss it with me. If I've forgotten anyone, it's due only to my memory loss and not because you haven't been wonderful.

You're holding this book in your hands today because of the amazing work of my tireless agent and dear friend Gina Panettieri, who believed in it and in me. Gina, I can't thank you enough for seeing how important this book is and for truly being there for me in every personal and professional crisis.

Acknowledgments

Thanks to my friends, Belle Wong and Brigitte Thompson who listen to me go on and on about whatever book I am currently working on. A very special thank you to my own incredible doctor, Maria Corigliano, M.D., who has seen me through my pregnancies with laughter, respect, honesty, thoughtfulness, and always a hug for good measure.

I wish I could find the words to express my love and thanks to my astounding husband, who was a complete partner in all of my pregnancies and is a complete partner in parenthood and life. And, of course, I have nothing but love for the results of my own pregnancies—my two wonderful children who truly make my world go round.

Introduction

Congratulations on your pregnancy! This book is written for all of the gorgeous, amazing, plus-size women who are out there creating beautiful babies. (That's you!)

Read this book as a supplement to your other pregnancy books. Your other pregnancy books will walk you through your baby's development, the changes in your body, and explanations of labor and delivery. Use those other books to get a broad overview of all pregnancy issues and topics. But then use this book as your complete guide to all the things those books don't tell plus-size moms that you've been wondering about or will come across during *your* pregnancy.

Your pregnancy is a wonderful, incredible thing and your body is beautiful and miraculous. We want this book to help you as you appreciate and enjoy that. Too often, plus-size women are made to feel like second-class citizens, and this problem is only worsened during pregnancy. During pregnancy, many women have to deal with health-care providers (doctors or midwives) who make them feel bad about their size, maternity-clothing manufacturers who don't get that we do need to wear maternity clothes and prefer not to look like a sack of potatoes in them, nurses who make a big deal out of finding the larger blood pressure cuff, hospital gowns that don't cover what they need to, and a perception by the media and some parts of the medical community that being plus size and pregnant is a dire condition that spells disaster.

All of that can really get you down and make you worry or feel terrible about yourself, just at the point in life when *any* size woman needs a lot of support and positive reinforcement. This book is here to help you celebrate the positives and cope with the negatives.

This is for all plus-sized women, from size 14 (or 12 depending on whose definition of plus size you use) to "super-size" (beyond size 24). Some of the problems and concerns discussed in this book impact different-sized women within this range—for example, some things might only be an issue for a woman who is a size 20 or smaller, while other things might apply only to larger women.

We've tried to include everyone and urge you to take the advice that you feel applies to you and your situation. We think ALL plus-size women are beautiful and deserve respect and support.

We wrote this book because the subject matter is near and dear to both of our hearts. Brette Sember is a plus-size mom of two who has experienced a seemingly unending labor, an unplanned C-section, a planned C-section, a miscarriage, PCOS, a very big baby, nursing and bottle-feeding. She's lost and gained weight and agonized over how much to gain and what to do when she couldn't seem to lose it. She's had exceptional health-care providers and health-care providers who made her feel two feet tall. She's felt good and bad about herself, her body and her pregnancies. Bruce D. Rodgers, M.D. is a Maternal-Fetal Medicine Specialist who works everyday with plus-size pregnant women and knows the joys and challenges as you work with your health-care provider through your pregnancy, delivery, and post-partume time. By combining our experiences and knowledge, we have tried to offer a thoughtful and balanced perspective on plus-size pregnancy that will help you experience a healthy and happy pregnancy.

You've probably read things in the media or had your own doctor talk to you about being plus size and pregnant. The goal of this book is to provide you with the solid medical facts and to explain them in a way that isn't anxiety inducing or frightening. It's also to help you see that your plus-size pregnancy is not a terrible medical condition, but is instead something for you to enjoy and appreciate.

This book is here to make you feel good about your amazing pregnancy, your gorgeous body, and ultimately, that wonderful baby you're growing. There are lots of books and magazine articles out there that will make you feel bad about yourself when it comes to your size. Often being overweight is just mentioned in passing in the mainstream pregnancy information, and when it's mentioned, it's made to sound like a serious problem. Well don't worry. There are no scare tactics here. *Your Plus-Size Pregnancy* is about looking at risks and concerns objectively in a calm and realistic way, while emphasizing how to feel good about yourself. We know that most women who are plus size and pregnant have healthy pregnancies and perfect babies, and this book is here to support you through your successes. This book is here to shout from the rooftops that you can have a healthy and wonderful pregnancy!

Throughout these pages, you will find quotes from real women. Hundreds of plus-size moms were interviewed for this book (some were even pregnant at the time of the interviews) and generously allowed us to include their thoughts and opinions. These quotes let you hear from lots of women in your shoes and get real advice from those in the trenches.

You'll also find statistics from medical studies about weight and pregnancy. This information is included so that you can have the cold, hard scientific facts, but we're not just throwing this information at you and letting you puzzle through it and hyperventilate over it. Our intent is to look seriously at what these statistics mean and in realistic terms. So, while a study might say plus-size women have twice the risk of average-weight women for a certain problem (and that does sound pretty scary), this means that if a normal weight woman has a 1-percent chance, then a plus-size woman has only a 2-percent chance. When you look at it in those terms, it doesn't sound so scary and is nothing to spend your nights worrying about. The intent of this book is not to downplay in any way the important research that's been done (and is still ongoing) about weight and pregnancy, but rather to present the information in a way that lets you understand it, work through it, make your own choices, and then move on with your life.

We also want to be clear that we're not saying, "Yippee, let's all go chow down on corn chips because weight doesn't matter when it comes to health and pregnancy." Of course weight matters (we know you know this), but so do a lot of other things. All women have some kind of risk in pregnancy. Some women smoke, some have family histories of Tay-Sachs disease, some have hormone irregularities, some have high blood pressure, some have asthma, some are underweight—the list goes on and on. You come to pregnancy with whom you are and work from there. It's always important that you talk with your own health-care provider to get advice about your own situation. A book is never a substitute for personal medical advice and we urge you to discuss your concerns and questions with your own health-care provider. We think you're terrific the way you are and are not here to lecture you, make you feel bad, or be the weight police. There's way too much of that now as it is. Our goal is to give you information, provide some realistic approaches to concerns you may have, help you focus on the positives, feel great about yourself, and include lots and lots of support.

Most importantly though, our goal is to help you approach your pregnancy with dignity, pride, comfort, and joy.

1

Loving Who You Are

he most wonderful thing in the world is happening to you! You're about to become a mother. If this is your first pregnancy, you are probably overwhelmed by the incredible miraculousness, yet sheer simplicity of how your body is doing this. It's almost beyond comprehension, yet it's so basic that your body knows how to do it without any help.

Pregnancy is an incredible time—there is so much anticipation and joy—yet it can also be a difficult time. Not only are you sick, tired, hormonal, and achy, but it can be hard to feel good about your changing body. This is especially difficult for many plus-size women because we have a long history of hating our bodies and feeling bad about ourselves. Now, more than ever, you need to find a way to feel good about your body and everything it is going through.

"The pressures that are put on women in our society to be perfect are completely unrealistic. You should strive to be the healthiest you that you can be. If that means a size 8 or 28, if you are happy and healthy, that is all that matters. You are beautiful."—Becky A.

"I believe there is something beautiful about every woman, plus sized or not. And nothing is more beautiful than a pregnant woman."—Ali S.

"I began to actually love my body for the first time when I was pregnant—instead of viewing it, my body, as a fat, ugly blob, it was a life-giving system, producing the most incredible miracle I would ever receive. I began to love it—really love it—for helping me give life to another."—Dana C.

"Just love your body. Because if you love your body, your kids will learn to love their bodies and that's really the most important thing. Our bodies may be larger than some, but they are also smaller than others. We are strong, capable, smart and able to have healthy pregnancies just as well as anyone else. Don't let anyone scare you!"—Liz O.

Liking Yourself

You may have struggled with weight issues your entire life, or you might have recently put on a few pounds. Either way, as your pregnancy care provider will tell you, and as you will learn in this book, *pregnancy is not the time to try to lose weight*. You have a baby to nurture, and you can't do that if you're starving yourself or yo-yo dieting. Pregnancy is a time when you must accept who you are for the sake of your baby and take your body as it is.

This time in your life is a time of selflessness. You're doing other things for your baby now—giving up certain medications, refusing a glass of wine, and gagging at the thought of celery. And you know that bigger sacrifices will come once the baby is born and your entire lifestyle changes. If you can accept these changes, and even embrace them (except for the gagging over celery), you can accept the fact that this is a time when you must accept your bodies as it is and stop agonizing over it.

It's time to find a way to love your body. It's time to see your body as a life-giving factory, one that is no better or no worse than anyone else's. And it's time to see the beauty in your shape. We've all been raised in a society where thin is better. But it's simply not true. Underweight women are at a high risk of delivering underweight babies, babies who are at risk for respiratory problems and bleeding in the brain. They also have difficulty conceiving. Smaller is definitely not better. There are benefits and detriments to every body size, and it's time to sit down and just accept what size you will be throughout this pregnancy.

"If the world were full of stick-thin people, we'd all look the same. A mob of sheep, basically. Thank goodness we are all different because that's what makes the world interesting. You're not a bad person because you're big, so don't ever let anyone tell you otherwise. I think you have to be philosophical about your size and learn to live with it and love yourself for the person you are. Unfortunately, the media sends out the very powerful message that you have to be stick thin to be a good or nice and successful person, and everyone aspires to be like A-List Hollywood stars. It's rubbish."—Sharon L.

"I have always been self-conscious about my weight, although I have been a size 6 and a size 26. Most days I have to remember that who I am begins with the love, respect, and confidence I have within myself. I am not the same person at either size spectrum, although I used to claim I was. So now my happiness is a renewal of spirit each day. That helps me stay focused and positive."—Cheryl H.

"We all have different set points or points at which our body is happy with its size. Did you know that women with 17 percent or less body fat have trouble conceiving children? True! So all those size 0 women have to have help making babies, and I would imagine pregnancy isn't a hayride for them either considering most aren't well-nourished enough to have anything to help nourish their babies. And they pass their freakish fanaticism about weight on to their daughters, if they have them, which is sad."—DeAnn R.

Body Image Acceptance

Knowing intellectually that your body is doing a great thing and looking at yourself in the mirror and feeling good are two different things. There are really three camps when it comes to body image. Take this quiz to find out which group you fall into:

When you stand in front of a mirror, you:
   A. have no problem looking at yourself
   B. focus on your face or clothing
   C. get away as quickly as possible

When someone compliments you on your appearance you:
   A. thank them graciously and feel good about the compliment
   B. brush it off and move on
   C. exclaim about how wrong they are

You're drinking a milkshake. You:
   A. enjoy every drop of it
   B. don't really think about calories while drinking it
   C. feel guilty with every sip

You're trying on clothes in a dressing room. You:
   A. take your time trying things on and choose clothing that is flattering to your figure and shows off your best parts
   B. try a few things on quickly and buy whatever fits
   C. become disgusted with how you look and leave the store without buying anything

If you answered with mostly *As*:
   You appreciate your body. You already see your own beauty and don't spend too much time agonizing over how you look or what other people think of you.

If you answered with mostly *Bs*:
   You avoid thinking about your body. You might avoid looking in the mirror or focus only on your face when confronted with a photo or

mirror image. You aren't happy about your weight, but you mostly push thoughts about it to the side.

If you answered with mostly *Cs*:

You can't stop thinking about your weight and really believe that you hate yourself and how you look. You might constantly be stepping on the scale or you might eat something and then feel terrible for hours about the calories you just ingested and promise yourself you'll eat less in the future.

If you're in group *A*, you've got a head start. You already understand that you are a beautiful woman and that beauty is about more than dress size or being able to compare yourself to the latest starving fashion model. You're on the right track!

If you're in group *B*, you're in denial about your body. Deep inside you don't like how you look, so you avoid thinking about it or dealing with it.

If you're in group *C*, you're actively engaged in self-hatred, and it's time to make a change. You can do this!

So, how do you start to accept yourself for who you are? How do you find a way to love your body through your pregnancy? How do you turn off the voice inside you that whispers unkind things?

Follow these tips:

1. Read Chapter 5, and talk to your doctor or midwife about weight gain during pregnancy so you fully and completely understand how important maintaining or gaining a certain amount is.

2. Remember that during your pregnancy, you are responsible for another human being's existence. Losing weight is just not a sensible option for you (unless your doctor or midwife tells you so).

3. Remember that ALL women get big during pregnancy. It is impossible to carry a healthy baby and not grow a belly and bigger breasts. Your body is supposed to change. The changes you will see are good, which means things are developing normally.

4. You gain nothing by beating yourself up about your body shape or size, so stop doing it. Telling yourself negative things is not going to make you feel any better.

5. Keep in mind that a scale only provides one small piece of information about you. It's easy to get too wrapped up in that number, since you're seeing it every time you go to the doctor during pregnancy, but you must know and must believe that it is only one fraction of who you are.

6. Force yourself to think positive, happy thoughts about your body and your self-image. If you think it, you will be it. Think of yourself as an attractive, happy, smart, adjusted person and you will radiate this image.

7. Avoid the things that are designed to make you feel bad. Recognize that much of our mainstream culture is designed to make people feel unworthy, unimportant, unattractive and just generally lacking. Don't read magazines with wafer-thin models in them. Don't watch reality shows that are all about changing people's appearances.

Separating Size from Self

If you hate or dislike being a plus-size woman, it's important that you learn to separate weight from identity. Who you are is not defined by your looks or weight. Who you are is defined by what you do, how you act, and how you feel. You have the choice of identifying yourself as a lawyer, wife, secretary, artist, gardener, or mother. You can identify yourself by your personal characteristics—artistic, kind, funny, intelligent, practical, organized, creative, friendly, and so on. If you choose to think of yourself as someone who is fat, ugly, too big, or not pretty, then that's what other people will see. It's up to you to define who you are and focus on being that person. Sure, society has some set expectations about what makes a person successful or attractive, but just as there are those expectations, there are plenty of people who are attractive or successful without starving themselves into a size 0.

Dr. Merry McVey-Noble, cognitive behavioral psychologist at the Bio-Behavioral Institute in Great Neck, New York, professor of psychology at Hofstra University and proud plus-size mom says, "Your body is yours, but it is not you. You are so much more than the sum of your parts. Becoming hooked on your appearance and the pursuit of perfection with regard to it is as dangerous as becoming hooked on a drug. Body obsessions are particularly pernicious because you have to live with your own body. Instead of treating it like an object and trying always to perfect it or control it, try accepting it." Dr. McVey-Noble suggests accepting each part of your body by itself instead of standing in front of the mirror and hating your entire self. Accepting one piece of your body at a time is much easier. "People will never dissect you like you do yourself," she says. "If you can accept you, others will."

"When you learn you are pregnant and you are large, you have no choice but to accept your size then and there. You are not allowed to diet! Somehow you have to figure out mentally that you will feel good about yourself, your pregnancy, and of course, your baby, and be excited about the new chapter in your life. In a way, hearing that you can't diet for nine months is a blessing because it removes that pressure. You can exercise, you can meditate, and of course, you can eat healthy things. If there was ever a time when I felt that my life was in the hands of the universe, it was when I was pregnant."—Liz R.

"I loved being pregnant, and it was one of the few times in my life that I haven't hated my size. I was much less self-conscious about the way I looked at it. It was like the pregnancy made it all right to be fat since I had a baby growing in there."—Carla R.

"The key to acceptance is asking yourself if you are healthy. Most of us would rather be thinner, but some of us are simply destined to be bigger women. As long as you are able to physically do all of the things you want to do, accept that you are beautiful no matter what your size."—Amelia M.

List 10 positive things about yourself:

1. _____
2. _____
3. _____
4. _____
5. _____
6. _____
7. _____
8. _____
9. _____
10. _____

These are the things about you that are important and valuable and define who you are. Focus on these things, instead of what you think of as negative things. Remind yourself what you're good at, and celebrate the parts of your body that you love.

Your Right to Be Pregnant and Enjoy It

Despite the fascination in our culture with being thin, there are many women who enjoy pregnancy thoroughly because it is a time to enjoy becoming more shapely. You have this right as much as anyone. Pregnancy is fleeting. While you're going through it, it might seem as if it lasts for eons, but in the whole scheme of your life, it's really just a small little moment. Because it will slip through your fingers so quickly, you must absolutely make the most of it or you will regret it.

Enjoying pregnancy doesn't mean eating everything you can get your hands on, though unfortunately there is a terrible stereotype that this is what larger women do. This may be why so many doctors feel compelled to lecture their plus-size patients early in pregnancy about not going overboard or not giving themselves license to be pigs. But pregnancy does mean you may be hungry more often and crave different things. You should listen to your hunger, your cravings, and your body. There really are very few large women who see pregnancy as an excuse to gain 100 pounds, as some health-care providers might fear. Pregnancy is not a time to deprive yourself, and eating in a sensible way does not have to mean depriving yourself.

You've probably seen pregnant celebrities wearing form-fitting or belly-baring clothes. There's no reason why you shouldn't choose clothing that accentuates your pregnant belly if you feel comfortable doing so. Enjoying and showing off that lovely bump is your prerogative. There's no reason to hide in a tent if you don't want to. Your pregnancy is just as beautiful as anyone else's, and the work your body is doing is admirable and important.

Enjoying your pregnancy is about more than just physical things, though. It's about taking the time to appreciate the hard work your body is doing. It's about feeling awe at your body's incredible intelligence. It's about reveling in the notion that an act of love made this baby (and even if you used a sperm donor or didn't plan this pregnancy, conceiving and choosing to have a baby was an act of love). You deserve to take the time to ease into your pregnancy. Rub your belly. Put up your feet. Have a glass of milk and a couple of cookies if you want. Show some of your newly defined cleavage. This is your pregnancy, and it's your special time. Enjoy every moment of it that you can, and don't let anyone stand in your way.

"Just have fun being pregnant—it's really a gift."—Liz R.

"I was self-conscious a little, but I loved everyone knowing I was pregnant. I rushed into maternity clothes and probably put on a few pounds early on in the pregnancy because I wanted the belly. I also loved being able to indulge in the foods that made me feel good and happy."—Vanessa R.

Taking Charge of Your Pregnancy

Although pregnancy is something your body is going to manage without any direction from you, the practical aspects of your pregnancy are up to you. Finding a health-care provider, choosing childbirth classes, buying maternity clothes, exercising, and developing a happy mind-set are all things that are within your control. Sometimes when you're trudging to doctor appointments and being poked and prodded or spending time hanging over the toilet in the mornings, it's easy to feel as though pregnancy is something that happens to you. But you own this pregnancy, and there are many decisions to be made that are yours alone. You're the captain of this pregnancy ship, and taking charge of it will help you feel in control and more positive.

It can be easy to feel as though your health-care provider is the one who's in charge. But he or she is there to give you information and advice. It's up to you to make decisions. Chapter 3 gives information about finding and working with a health-care provider.

The best way to feel good about your pregnancy is to control its course. If you go to doctor appointments or to maternity stores feeling as if other people know better than you do what will work best for you,

you are giving up control. This is your baby, and you're the only one who can make decisions about him or her. And one of the most important decisions you must make is that you will love yourself and your pregnancy.

Decide today—right now—that you are proud and happy to be a plus-size pregnant woman, and that from today forward, you will be the one who decides how you will be cared for, looked at, talked about, and supported.

2

Dealing with Your Changing Body

*P*regnancy is a time of great change. You're on the cusp of a huge lifestyle change (soon you'll be a mom!), and you're experiencing incredible physical and emotional upheaval. Some people think that the changes that pregnancy brings are nature's way of preparing you for the changes the baby will bring. All pregnant women struggle to deal with the sometimes overwhelming experiences of gestation. And plus-size moms in particular may struggle with the transformation pregnancy brings to their bodies. While it might seem at times that the changes are too much, you will be able to manage them. This chapter will look at some of the most common changes or problems you may encounter during your pregnancy. Everyone's body is different, and everyone reacts differently to pregnancy. If you have concerns about symptoms you're experiencing, talk to your health-care provider.

While you're getting used to your changing body, you'll also have to deal with the lunacy pregnancy can bring. Buckle up for a roller-coaster ride of joy, terror, anticipation, weepiness, anxiousness, exuberance, excitement, and impatience. Your pregnancy is sure to bring with it a wide array of emotions, many of which will be unpredictable. It's hard enough to deal with physical changes, but emotional changes can sometimes sneak up on you unexpectedly.

Dr. McVey-Noble points out, "Our bodies were never meant to stay the same forever. Whatever changes occur that don't have catastrophic or lethal consequences, welcome them. Say, 'Thank God I'm OK!' and realize that your body and all of its scars or stretch marks and other imperfections tell the story of your life."

Coping with Weight Gain

Weight gain is an important part of pregnancy. Chapter 5 discusses what a healthy amount of weight to gain is, and it is important to talk with your doctor about your individual situation. If you do gain weight during your pregnancy (and most women should gain at least some), it might be hard to reconcile yourself to the idea. If you've spent years trying to lose weight, it can be quite difficult to suddenly accept the fact that weight gain is now a good thing. It can be particularly hard to step on a scale and see the numbers go up and think, "Well, there's another pound I'm going to have to try to lose after the baby comes."

If you're nervous about gaining too much weight, worried about how to lose weight after the birth, or disgusted at the thought of gaining weight, this can be a difficult time for you. The first thing you must do is look at this with a clinical eye. You are growing a baby inside you, and the baby needs nourishment. Your body is going to provide it, and to do so, you must gain some weight. When you gain weight during pregnancy, it is not about some personality flaw or control issue. You're providing a healthy environment for your baby to grow in.

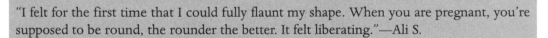

According to the March of Dimes, this is the breakdown of where weight gain goes during pregnancy:

Baby: about 7.5 pounds (depending on your baby's size)

Blood: 3 pounds

Breasts: 2 pounds

Uterus: 2 pounds

Placenta: 1.5 pounds

Amniotic fluid: 2 pounds

Fat, protein, and other nutrients: 7 pounds

Retained water: 7 pounds

You shouldn't feel guilty about gaining weight or worry what people will think. As long as you and your health-care provider are satisfied with where your weight is, you can remind yourself that you're doing exactly what you're supposed to be doing. And gaining only the recommended amount can make it easier to take pregnancy weight off once the baby comes.

"If you're eating healthy, you can't look at the numbers. Your body is doing what's best for the baby, so just watch the snacks and try to do the best you can."—Lisa B.

"I felt for the first time that I could fully flaunt my shape. When you are pregnant, you're supposed to be round, the rounder the better. It felt liberating."—Ali S.

"The only thing I did not like was that my stomach was too fat for my tummy button to pop out."—Rachel G.

Nausea

Your weight has no link to nausea, so don't worry that the reason you're feeling so sick has to do with your weight. If you experience morning sickness, don't worry if you actually lose some weight at the beginning of your pregnancy. Always discuss a drop in weight with your health-care provider, but know that this is a very common effect of nausea.

There are probably as many ways to fight nausea as there are pregnant women. Many women swear by dry crackers, eating more protein, or eating more fat. There is no one solution that works for everyone. If you find that your prenatal vitamin is bothering you, take it later in the day or with a meal, or ask your health-care provider about switching brands. Open windows, or turn on exhaust fans to remove food smells from your kitchen or home.

To help reduce nausea, try eating small meals every three hours. Eating before you are hungry might circumvent nausea. Consider eating only cold food or foods that are easily digestible. Stay away from greasy or spicy foods or any other food that just makes you feel sick. Increase your fluid intake, and stay hydrated at all times. If nothing else works, talk to your health-care provider about taking a vitamin B-6 supplement. Iron can sometimes upset your stomach, so talk to your health-care provider about the iron content in your vitamin.

Some over-the-counter remedies might work for you—Sea Band motion sickness bracelets work on pressure points, and Preggie Pops lollipops have ingredients that are soothing to your stomach. Ginger and peppermint can work to reduce morning sickness, so try teas or lozenges in these flavors.

Avoid hot rooms or warm places since getting overheated can make morning sickness worse. Avoid aromas that bother you, and if you find you're really sensitive to smells, carry something that you can sniff instead. Getting enough sleep can help reduce morning sickness.

"In the hospital they introduced me to the 'wet-dry' diet. This is a two-day diet designed to reset the body since sometimes nausea and vomiting can become cyclic. All this entails is that you don't take in fluids with your meals. You eat your meal—dry— and then wait I think an hour or two and then have your fluids—wet. Wet things include soup, drinks, ice cream, etc. They also recommended consuming protein when nauseated, which I wouldn't have considered on my own. But they were right. I found that eggs—

shockingly enough—were my friend when it came to warding off serious nausea. So was just the meat from a hamburger."—Michelle C.

"Preggie Pops! The ginger ones really help with nausea."—Becky A.

"The trick that worked for me was to eat protein just before bed. I would curl up a few pieces of lunch meat (which didn't sound good at ALL) or cheese and gobble them in a few bites that way. The next morning, I'd awake nausea free."—Jeannie T.

"I used Sea Bands that fit on your wrist and apply pressure to the inside of your wrist. I wore them every day in the beginning, and they seemed to help a little."—Beth T.

"Ginger—this was a lifesaver for me. Real ginger tea, not ginger ale. Just slice up some ginger, and let it boil in some water for five or six minutes. You can add honey or lemon to better the taste. I kept ginger tea in my fridge at all times when I was first pregnant. Any hint of nausea and I would just take a couple sips of ginger tea, and I almost always felt better."—Joan T.

"I kept Saltines by the bed along with a glass of water. When I woke up, I would eat a few crackers while still in bed and have a few sips of water. This would help me avoid the nausea first thing in the morning."—Beth U.

"Never let yourself get hungry. That was always a big nausea trigger."—Liz O.

Yeast Infections

Hormonal changes during pregnancy make your body more prone to yeast infections. Being overweight predisposes many women to yeast infections because of high sugar content in their diet or because the size of their bodies decreases airflow in the vaginal region.

There are many over-the-counter treatments available, but if you've never had a yeast infection, it's important to get it diagnosed by your health-care provider before treating it since it could be something else. Also check with your health-care provider to be sure he or she feels over-the-counter treatments are safe during pregnancy. To prevent yeast infections, try to control your sugar intake and eat yogurt or take aci-dophilus supplements. Wear breathable panties, and try to find a time each day when you can sit with your legs apart to maximize airflow, especially if you tend to sit with your legs crossed or tightly together.

It's important to note that recurring yeast infections may be a symptom of gestational diabetes. So it is essential to talk with your health-care provider about yeast infections you experience during preg-nancy.

Heartburn

Being overweight is thought to increase your susceptibility to heartburn during pregnancy, although since 50 percent of women report some heartburn during pregnancy, you shouldn't feel as if your weight is the reason for it. Heartburn is usually common late in pregnancy when the size of the uterus presses on the stomach. If you're one of the "lucky" women who has to deal with heartburn during pregnancy, don't believe the old wives' tale that it has to do with the amount of the baby's hair—that hasn't been proven to be true, although lots of women insist it was the case for them.

The best way to cope with heartburn is to look at what you're eat-ing and when you're eating it. Avoid eating before lying down. Try eat-ing smaller, more frequent meals instead of large meals at one sitting. Avoid overeating since it will increase stomach acid. If there are certain foods you can tie directly to heartburn, eliminate them. Greasy foods might also be a cause. Caffeine can cause heartburn. Eating a small amount of yogurt or milk or taking a spoonful of honey dissolved in a glass of warm water can ease heartburn. Heartburn during pregnancy tends to get worse at night. If you're having problems in the night, try raising the head of your bed.

A recent study in the medical journal *Gut* showed that people who regularly add salt to their food are 70 percent more likely to have acid reflux, or heartburn. Cutting back on salt may be another way to reduce problems with heartburn.

Unfortunately, sometimes there doesn't seem to be any direct correlation between heartburn and what you eat or when you eat it. An over-the-counter antacid like Tums or Rolaids is a good solution. They come in a variety of flavors, so you can probably find one you like. Avoid antacids that contain sodium, which can increase fluid buildup. Taking an antacid one hour after meals and at bedtime may help reduce your discomfort.

Some cases of heartburn are caused by gastroesophageal reflux disease (GERD). If you have GERD, you can probably expect it to get worse during pregnancy. Treatment for GERD includes removing nicotine and caffeine, avoiding greasy or highly acidic foods, as well as all of the previously mentioned tips. There are prescription medications that are used to treat GERD during pregnancy, so talk to your health-care provider if you have GERD.

"I had Tums stashed in the car, my purse, my pockets, everywhere to help with the seemingly constant heartburn towards the end of the pregnancy."—Beth U.

Constipation

Constipation is one of the unpleasant side effects of pregnancy. If you had constipation problems before pregnancy, you can probably expect them to continue. If you've never had a problem, you may now. To reduce constipation, avoid caffeine and drink more water. Eat foods that are high in fiber, and make dietary changes to increase fiber in your diet, such as eating more fruit or switching from white bread to wheat bread or from white rice to brown rice. If you have an ongoing problem with constipation, you can take a fiber supplement. Iron supplements can lead to constipation, so talk to your health-care provider about your vitamins. Physical activity can also help with constipation—moving your body gets your intestines moving. Never take a laxative without first asking your health-care provider.

"I had to up my fiber intake during pregnancy to prevent constipation."—Lee T.

Coping with Aches and Pains

Oh, the aches and pains of pregnancy. Sometimes you feel as though your body is just not going to make it through another day—or another night. You can't get comfortable standing, sitting, or lying down. Pregnancy can be uncomfortable no matter what your size.

There are some solutions that can help keep you more comfortable. Sit in chairs that offer good upright back support, or get a lumbar support pillow to put behind you. Put your feet up when possible. If you work in an office, think about bringing in a small footstool to put under your desk so you can put your feet up while you work. Avoid chairs with arms if you find you don't fit comfortably. Remember to put your seat belt underneath your belly and not over it. Don't be afraid to ask for a seat-belt extension if you fly on an airplane. If you don't fit comfortably in an airplane seat, make sure your traveling companion is seated next to you, and put up the armrest between you. Adjust the seat in your car to provide more back support or change the angle of the seat to make yourself more comfortable.

Moving around or changing positions will help you feel more comfortable. Wear comfortable shoes, even if you have to sacrifice fashion for comfort. Nice warm baths or hot showers can be a terrific cure-all for general soreness and tiredness.

Do gentle stretches to loosen up your muscles and learn specific stretches for your most painful areas. (See the Appendix for links or ask your health-care provider.) Attending a pregnancy exercise class can be a lifesaver if you can't figure out what to stretch or how to stretch it. You might also want to buy a pregnancy-exercise tape and try doing some of the stretches in it. Sometimes larger women have weaker abdominal muscles, and the extra weight of a baby can cause lower-back or round-ligament pain. Pregnancy Pilates exercise videos or classes may help you strengthen these muscle groups and stay more comfortable.

If you are having a lot of lower-back or round-ligament pain, consider buying a pregnancy belly support. This elastic belt goes underneath your belly and helps to hold it up. Some have straps that go over your shoulders to more evenly distribute the weight burden. If you do buy one (see Chapter 9 for more information about purchasing), remember that you might grow so accustomed to it that you will feel very uncomfortable without it.

If you are having difficulty crossing your legs or are experiencing a lot of varicose veins, you may need to find new ways to sit. Crossing an ankle over the other knee is a good alternative to regular leg crossing because it doesn't put as much pressure on your legs. Sitting with your legs crossed just down at the ankles can give you the feeling of being ladylike without the discomfort. Also, sitting straight up in a chair with both feet planted on the ground next to each other can be a very comfortable (and posture-friendly) position.

Staying active during pregnancy can help keep you comfortable. Even if you just do some stretching at home (see Appendix) or walk for exercise, this may be enough to keep things flexible. Don't do exercises or stretches if they make you hurt more!

The key to relieving discomfort is understanding what is causing it. Your office chair or high heels might be the cause of your back pain, but until you pinpoint this, you aren't going to be able to do anything to make it better. Talk to your health-care provider about any aches and pains you have, and see if she or he can help you get to the bottom of them. Bottom line, though, sometimes pregnancy itself is just uncomfortable, and you have to get through it as best you can. This is not the time in your life to prove how tough you are. It's a time to take it easy on yourself. Don't be afraid to sit more often or elevate your legs if it makes you feel even slightly better.

An important note is that if you are in pain, you should discuss it with your health-care provider. ALL women have discomfort during pregnancy. Your health-care provider can put you on disability leave if you are not able to comfortably do your job (if you can't stand or sit as you need to for your job), so don't be afraid to ask about it.

"If you have to stand for a long time, try alternating your feet by putting one on a small step stool and then switching to alternate the pressure."—Angie G.

"I do believe there is a lot more discomfort for heavy women, one because of size and adding even more, and usually babies are bigger. I did have a lot of discomforts, but you need to learn what helps to ease them. Put your feet up as much as possible to help with swelling."—Jennifer

"Don't sit too long. Get up and move around every so often so that the circulation gets to move in your backside and lower limbs."—Sharon L.

"Backrubs by my husband made all the difference in the world."—Jennifer H.

"I suffered sciatica from the third month of my second pregnancy, and it was very apparent when I was standing. It became uncomfortable to stand for long periods, and walking was difficult at times."—Sharon L.

"I have pain in my lower back and low in my pelvic area, and pelvic rocks (which are recommended) only make it worse. A lumbar pillow and using the lumbar support in the car are very helpful."—Merry M.

"I bought an overstuffed, big office chair and a footrest and used that while working at the office."—DeAnn R.

"My biggest problem was that I drive a Jeep and had to have the seat taken out and moved back."—Tammy M.

"To help with the discomfort, I used a heating pad on my back at night."—Beth U.

"Hot showers take almost every ailment away. When doing dishes, I would open the cupboard and put my foot inside it. It took the pressure off my back. Computer work was excruciating sometimes, so I'd get up every twenty minutes and stretch or walk around."—Amelia M.

Sleeping

Once the baby comes, sleep is going to be at a premium, but somehow your body doesn't seem to understand how much you need to stock up on sleep now! You might find it's impossible to get comfortable, or you might be making so many trips to the bathroom during the night that you just can't get any solid sleep.

If you find yourself going to the bathroom a lot at night, reduce your fluid intake in the evening. Drink more during the rest of the day so that your bladder won't get as full at night. Install a night-light in your bathroom so that you don't need to turn on the light when you're in there, which only serves to wake you up more fully.

Body pillows are the absolute answer to nighttime discomfort. (See Appendix for links.) There is a wide variety of choices available, so shop around, and choose a brand and style that seems best suited to you. Friends who have had babies may still have their old pillows, and you can borrow those or use them to test different styles.

Some women don't use body pillows and use several regular pillows instead. This can allow you to get the support you need at just the right place, but may mean you need to make more adjustments during the night. The key to comfortable sleep is a pillow between your legs, if at all possible. Try different size pillows until you hit upon the right one.

If you're sick and tired of sleeping on your side, put a pillow underneath one hip and that side of your back, so you are slightly tipped to the side, and lay on your back. You will still avoid putting too much pressure on the inferior vena cava (a vein which can reduce blood flow to the placenta if you put pressure on it) and enjoy being able to sleep in a slightly different position.

If you are feeling discomfort from your stomach pulling down to the side while you're lying on your side, put a small pillow underneath that side of your belly to give it some support. This will reduce the pulling you might feel on your abdomen. You might also find that you need to wear a bra to bed to keep your breasts in a comfortable position.

"Get a body pillow to support your weight while you sleep. This makes the last trimester so much more comfortable."—Ali S.

"Buy one of those really large, long pillows. I would drape my leg over it when I was on my side to raise the top hip up, otherwise my hips felt a lot of pressure."—Lisa B.

"Sleep on your side with a pillow under your feet and one between your legs and one behind your back."—Rachel G.

"Babies 'R' Us has a terrific wrap pillow, like a big C, which is awesome. Tuck the bottom part between your knees, it supports your back and is cozy to snuggle. The top wraps from under your head down in front of you."—Vanessa R.

"At one time, my husband threatened to sleep on the lounge. He had to fight for space in the bed because I had five pillows: behind my back, under my belly, between my legs, and two under my head, supporting me."—Sharon L.

"A cool mist humidifier is wonderful for sleeping since pregnancy makes your nose stuffy."—Jennifer W.

Shape Change

Even at the beginning of pregnancy you will probably notice changes in your body. For many women, the first change they notice is larger breasts. You might also suddenly look rounder, even though you're not really "showing." Just because you are plus sized doesn't mean that pregnancy will not immediately affect your shape. In fact, seeing that shape change in the beginning can be very encouraging and help you feel really pregnant. Some women report few noticeable shape changes in the beginning of their pregnancies. If this is you, you shouldn't feel bad about it or be worried. You're still just as pregnant as any other woman, and your baby is developing just as well.

If you do experience breast changes, you may need to purchase a maternity bra or simply a larger size. It can be helpful to get measured or at least to try on a few different sizes before making a purchase. If your breasts get larger, they might be sore, and having good support will help ease discomfort.

"Get a really good supportive bra, and don't skimp on a good one."—Lisa B.

"[My breasts] got bigger fast. I just made sure to keep lotion on them and made sure that my husband was gentle anytime he came in contact with them. He liked that they got bigger."—Vanessa R.

"The biggest tip I'd give someone with aching breasts is to keep your bra on when you can or get a sport bra to make you more comfortable."—Jill G.

"I liked my clearly larger and rounder breasts."—Jen R.

"Enjoy it, and show them off. It's the only part of a woman's body that society likes to get bigger."—Amelia M.

Sex

Now that you're pregnant, sex is no longer for baby-making, but is perfect for fun, love, and comfort. Continuing to have a healthy sex life will be important for you and your partner, as long as your health-care provider gives you the green light. Some plus-size moms report feeling uncomfortable about their growing bodies and unable to enjoy sex, but many are able to focus on their budding bodies or on their partners and get beyond any negative feelings. You may find that sex relaxes you and de-stresses you. It can also allow you and your partner to feel close to each other at a time when many things in your lives are changing.

Your partner loved your prepregnancy body, and he will love your pregnant and postnatal body, also. The biggest obstacle to enjoying sex during pregnancy is often mental. If you're having trouble believing that he still likes your body, talk about your feelings. In most cases, he will be able to reassure you that you are still sexy.

Finding a comfortable position during sex can be challenging, especially in the last trimester. Many women interviewed for this book reported enjoying being on top or being on their hands and knees with their partner behind them. Spooning may also be an alternative to consider. Read some books, such as *The Pregnancy Bible* or *Hot Mamas* (see Appendix) for photos/illustrations and directions for different positions. Some women report having an increased desire during pregnancy, while others find they are less interested than ever before—and you might experience both at different times.

If you're feeling self-conscious about your body, remind yourself that your partner is happy about the reason it's changing and knows the important work it's doing. And above all, it's just temporary. After the baby comes, you can slowly get back to normal. If you are feeling really uncomfortable, consider making love wearing a pretty or sexy nightgown, under the covers, or with the lights off. The best bet is to tell your partner how you're feeling and get his input. You'll probably be happy to learn he finds your pregnant body exciting and beautiful.

"On top is best because you have the control, which is always nice, and your belly doesn't get in the way."—Ali S.

"Be the one on top—it's easier, but for me it wasn't comfortable for long because of the leg position."—Lisa B.

"Doggy style works best."—Rachel G.

"My husband had no qualms about pregnant sex. He liked not having to use protection! Toward the end, the last month or so, it was sometimes awkward, but we made a point to make love often. We wanted it to induce labor."—Vanessa R.

"It's so important not to let this part of your relationship with your spouse fall apart. It helps remind you that you are still a couple, not just parents."—Beth U.

"Don't let a bigger belly put you off. A good orgasm is so relaxing." Melissa S.

"Sex became really different and in a very good way, so enjoy it, don't be afraid of it." —Jennifer V.

"After about month five, I wasn't really comfortable with sex, so my husband had to be satisfied with oral sex, which he was."—DeAnn R.

"Talk to your partner about how your pregnancy may affect sexual relations, and ask for his understanding if your libido takes a dive."—Sharon L.

"I was surprised that my sex drive increased, especially during the second trimester. My husband really liked when we would even just snuggle since it would give him an excuse to pat or talk to my naked belly."—Carla R.

"The doctor has prohibited me from engaging in sex for the remainder of my pregnancy. This at first made me feel very inadequate and unattractive. Cuddling and spending time with my hubby helped."—Richelle H.

"Admit that you feel unsexy, that's OK. Tell your mate that you need a lot of positive reinforcement about your femininity."—Amelia M.

Feeling the Baby Move

Some plus-size women feel their baby move a bit later than other women. There are a lot of factors other than weight involved in feeling those first movements (such as placement of the placenta). Most average women report feeling the baby move between sixteen and twenty weeks, although women who have already had a baby often can detect movement earlier because they know what it feels like. As long as your health-care provider is picking up a heartbeat and is not concerned, you have no reason to be concerned, either.

Some plus-size moms report that it was harder to see the baby's movements from the outside in the last trimester than it seemed with thinner people they know.

"With my first baby, around eighteen weeks, but with my second baby, I felt her move by twelve weeks. With my second, I saw her jumping from hiccups, rolling over, etc. So even if you are plus sized, these things can and will happen, just like everyone else."—Jennifer V.

3

Working with Your Health-Care Provider

*Y*our pregnancy health-care provider (usually a doctor or midwife) has a strong influence on the way you think about your pregnancy, feel about yourself, approach your health management, and your entire pregnancy and birth experience. It is essential that you find a doctor or health-care provider you like, can communicate with, and who treats you with kindness, respect, and a willingness to share information.

Going through a pregnancy with a health-care provider who makes you uncomfortable or nervous can make your entire pregnancy uncomfortable and unpleasant. But going through a pregnancy with a health-care provider you trust, respect, and like can be a joyous and wonderful experience.

It is possible to have a relaxed and comfortable relationship with your health-care provider. Sure, doctors and midwives are all about being healthy and you're overweight, but that doesn't mean that you and your health-care provider can't work together in a way that makes you comfortable while letting the doctor or midwife keep an eye on your health.

Size Acceptance

One of the most important issues facing a plus-size woman when selecting a pregnancy health-care provider is size acceptance. Consider these two scenarios:

Scenario #1:

The nurse or aide weighs you in the hallway with other patients and staff around. She starts with the weight at the 100-pound mark and then slowly and painstakingly moves the weights until she gets to your weight. She shakes her head as she records the information on your chart. She says, "You're up five pounds since last month." When you get to the exam room, she asks you to roll up your sleeve and then tightly wraps the regular-size blood-pressure cuff around your arm. It squeezes so hard you can barely stand it. You're relieved you don't have to take off your clothes because you remember that the gown was too small the last time. When the doctor comes in, she looks at the chart and says, "You've gained too much weight already. You have to stop eating so much." She then tells you to go for a gestational diabetes test because your weight puts you at a higher risk. You lay back for the exam, and she feels your tummy to check the baby. As you lie on your back with your shirt lifted up and your pants pulled partway down, she tells you "You're going to have a hard time delivering this one unless you get some exercise. You started this pregnancy overweight, and you don't need to gain nearly as much weight as normal women." You struggle to sit up and adjust your clothes. Before she leaves the room, she reminds you again to try to keep the weight in check.

Scenario #2:

The aide takes you back to a scale that is in a private alcove. The digital readout shows her your weight, and she records it. She makes pleasant chitchat with you. You go to the exam room, and she slips on a blood-pressure cuff that is comfortable and fits well. You don't need a gown, but remember that the last time you put on a gown, it fit comfortably. When the doctor comes in, he checks your chart and says "You're looking great. It's good that you're gaining some weight—it's important for the baby. I'd like to see you stay around a twenty-pound total gain if possible." He then asks you about how you feel, if you're staying active and if you have any questions. He checks the baby's size and position and gives you a hand to help pull yourself up after the exam. He reminds you that this month you're due for a gestational diabetes test and explains that they always check it at this point in the pregnancy. He mentions that you are at a slightly higher risk because of your weight, but that they test everyone. Before he leaves, he smiles and tells you that everything is progressing well and you're doing just fine.

Which experience would you rather have? It's pretty obvious! The first doctor may be an excellent physician, but she is not attuned to your feelings, emotions, and situation. The second doctor conveys the same information, but in a way that respects your feelings and intelligence. The first doctor might be a perfectly nice person and other women might adore her, but if she makes it clear that she disapproves of your size, it's not possible for you to feel comfortable with her.

You want to find a health-care provider who is size-accepting or size-friendly. This simply means the health-care provider and staff are sensitive to the feelings of plus-size patients. More and more doctors are becoming sensitive about how traditional medical care can make some women feel insulted, lectured to, or demeaned. A size-accepting doctor is sure to give you all the information and care you need, but does so in an atmosphere that does not make you feel like a child being scolded. He or she does not make a huge issue of your weight, accepts that you are who you are, and knows that you deserve to be treated with respect. The office staff maintains the same attitude.

"Find a size-positive, unprejudiced doc to care for you. And be specific when you go see them that you do NOT wish to be harangued about your size, as you know that pregnancy is not an appropriate time to diet."—DeAnn R.

"The best thing I did before I met with my doctor was to call and ask the staff about how they dealt with overweight/plus-size clients. They were really sweet, telling me some of them were "fluffy" themselves. They had some bigger gowns. I felt so much more comfortable having addressed the issue over the phone."—Tammy M.

Finding a Health-Care Provider

To find a doctor or provider, start by asking another provider you like for a referral. Ask friends and family for doctors or providers they recommend. If you are limited by your insurance policy as to which doctors you can see, obtain the list of approved providers. You can also use the American College of Obstetricians and Gynecologists "Find an Ob-Gyn" service on their Web site at *www.acog.org*.

Many people are hesitant to interview health-care providers, but you need to remember that this is your body, your baby, and your money paying for this provider. You are entitled to find out if you will feel comfortable with him or her.

Call the office, and ask point-blank if the doctor or midwife is size-friendly. The receptionist may not have a clue what you mean. This doesn't mean the provider is not size-friendly, it just means the receptionist has never had someone ask her that or that she is new. If the receptionist says "Yes," you know you're on the right track. If she doesn't know, let it go for now. Get the answers to your other questions, and if it seems that the provider meets most of your requirements, schedule a consultation. Usually this will take place in the office or exam room and will be relatively brief. Ask the provider about her attitude towards plus-size women. Watch her face and body for reactions. If she looks you in the eye, smiles, seems comfortable and confident, and gives you an answer you are happy with, you're probably on the right track. If your provider is a larger woman herself, it's not a guarantee she will be size-friendly. In fact, she might be even less friendly, with an attitude of "I know what it's like so I can be tough on you."

Ask if the office has large-size gowns and blood-pressure cuffs. Ask if your care will be different because you are larger. Ask if he stresses limiting weight gain when caring for patients or if he tries to be more relaxed about it. Find out what his position is on gestational diabetes tests. Some doctors feel that larger women need to be tested more often, even when they experience no problems. Explain that you are looking for a health-care provider you can feel comfortable with and are trying to get a feel for her approach.

In addition to size acceptance, you probably have other criteria for your health-care provider. Some factors may be more important to you than others. For example, a provider's age, race, or sex may be a matter of personal preference, while using a provider who is board certified and experienced working with plus-size moms should be a concern to all women. When you go to your first appointment, weigh the importance of, make note of, or ask the following:

- The provider's sex
- The provider's age
- His or her race
- Board certification
- Experience working with plus-size pregnant women

- How long he or she has been practicing medicine
- Whether there are other practitioners in the group
- Location
- Cost
- Insurance accepted
- How easy it is to schedule appointments at convenient times
- Average office waiting time
- Where he or she will deliver babies
- Openness to your birth-plan choices
- Caesarean (C-section) rate
- Episiotomy rate
- Forceps rate
- Office hours
- Whether children and/or partners are welcome at appointments

It is also important that you choose a health-care provider who has a high-risk pregnancy specialist (called a maternal-fetal medicine specialist) with whom he/she co-manages high-risk pregnancies. Because there is a slightly higher risk of some pregnancy complications for plus-size moms, you want a provider who is able to immediately hand your case over to, or consult with, a specialist if there is a problem.

Additionally, you need to ask your provider about the sophistication and quality of the ultrasound that is used in the office or at the facility where patients are referred. There can be difficulties in getting good-quality ultrasound results in plus-size women, so a more technically advanced machine may be necessary.

Ask at which hospital the provider delivers or refers patients and the quality and experience of the obstetrical anesthesiologists there, particularly when it comes to epidurals and intubation (insertion of breathing tubes for general anesthetic, see Chapter 14 for more information about this) experience with larger-size women. Find out which high-risk pregnancy center (level III hospital or regional perinatal center) the provider sends patients to if there is a problem.

You may also want to ask the provider if she routinely tests overweight women for gestational diabetes more often than women of other sizes and if so, how often. Some providers insist on testing frequently when this is not necessary. Ask the provider if your weight will have an impact on your care and if so, how.

If you select a provider and then realize you are not comfortable with him, you have the absolute right to leave and switch to a new provider. But keep in mind that most prefer not to accept women who are past the twenty-week mark in the pregnancy. If you're going to switch, do so in the first trimester, if possible. Remember that you are in control of your body and the medical treatment you receive. You can say no to any procedure, test, exam, doctor, health-care provider, or situation that makes you uncomfortable at any time.

"I started seeing my OB before I was pregnant, and she is also a large woman. When I became pregnant, I knew I would be comfortable with her because she is sensitive to size issues, the office has larger blood-pressure cuffs, and they never make a big deal out of weighing you."—Lee T.

"Just be frank and ask the important questions. Has this doctor worked with overweight pregnancies? Has the ultrasound tech worked with them? If there is a C-section needed, what kind of incision do you make and what precautions to prevent infection do you take, like a drain or higher incision? Is the office and hospital equipped with larger cuffs and gowns? That kind of thing. You should be comfortable there and not dread squeezing into a gown or getting an inaccurate BP that may affect your care."—Jen R.

What to Look for in the Office
There are some clues throughout the office that will help you get a feel for how size-friendly the health-care provider is.

Look to see where the scale is

A scale that is in a semiprivate location is best. No one wants to be weighed in a busy hallway or waiting room. A digital scale is a plus because you don't have to stand there for that endless adjustment of the little weights, and it can accommodate women whose weight might not register on the manual scales.

Notice the type of blood-pressure cuff used

If the office has a larger-size cuff (one is called a large cuff and the next size is a thigh cuff), notice if it is a big ordeal for the aide to go get it or whether it's done without comment. The best providers will have it ready. It is *very* important that your care provider use the right size cuff for your arm. Using smaller cuffs can give a false high blood-pressure reading.

Pay attention to the staff in the office

Are any of them large-sized? Are they friendly to you? Do you feel comfortable and treated with dignity while you are there?

Is the waiting room comfortable

Are other patients in the office larger sized? Are the chairs in the waiting room comfortable for your body? If you're not comfortable in the chair at the beginning of your pregnancy, you're definitely not going to be at the end of your pregnancy.

Make note of the gown you are given

Most offices have gowns of different sizes, but these often only go up to XL (which may not even fit a woman who is a true-size XL). If you are given a gown that is skimpy or uncomfortable, ask for another that will make you feel covered.

"I always ask for a thigh cuff when nurses go to take my blood pressure because I know that otherwise, they won't get an accurate reading. Regular-size cuffs on a larger person can make your blood pressure appear to be high when it isn't."—DeAnn R.

Midwives

You may choose to use a midwife as your primary pregnancy health-care provider, and nothing about being plus sized prevents you from considering this option. Some women have found that midwives can be more size accepting than M.D.s, and there are many other reasons why you might feel a midwife is the best provider for you.

Some midwives are on staff at an Ob/Gyn practice, while others work in a separate midwife practice. If you use a midwife, you may have the option of giving birth at home or at a birthing center where you may feel more comfortable and have more privacy.

If you are considering a midwife, you will want to ask the questions posed earlier in the chapter, but you also need to find out who the backup physician is for the midwife, should there be a problem during pregnancy or delivery. Ask about the backup physician's credentials and if he or she has experience working with plus-size patients.

To find a midwife, contact:

The American College of Nurse Midwives
www.acnm.org
240-485-1800

Midwives Alliance of North America
www.mana.org
888-923-MANA (6262)

North American Registry of Midwives
www.narm.org
888-842-4784

Talking to Your Provider About Weight

Once you find a provider you are comfortable with, you will have many questions about your pregnancy that you would like to have answered. Some of those questions will be about weight.

Questions to Ask About Weight

- How much weight gain do you recommend for me?
- Can you break that down by month or week for me?
- What happens if I gain too much in one or several months? Do I then have to try not to gain any more in later months?
- Should I try not to gain any weight at all?
- Am I at a higher risk for gestational diabetes, preeclampsia, still-birth, miscarriage, or C-section because of my weight? What can I do to reduce these risks?
- Does my weight place me at risk for other conditions or problems?
- What kind of exercise do you recommend for me?
- Should I try to eat more frequently during the day?
- Do you recommend seeing a nutritionist?
- Is the hospital/birth center size-friendly? Do they have gowns, blood-pressure cuffs, and abdominal supports that fit my size? If not, can you make sure they do?
- Will my size affect the baby?
- Will my size impact the baby's birth weight?
- What other things do I need to be aware of with regard to my weight?

Make sure you take the time to talk to your provider about the many other questions you have about pregnancy and birth that are not weight related.

Don't feel embarrassed or afraid to ask your provider any kind of question. He is there to serve your needs. You have the right to have your questions taken seriously and answered with complete explanations. If you don't feel you have enough information, ask for more. Remember to ask questions about weight or size without being timid or acting embarrassed. Asking questions about your health is an intelligent and rational thing to do. Being a beautiful plus-size pregnant woman is nothing to be ashamed or embarrassed about. You have the same right as any other woman to good medical care, and in order to get it, you need to be able to voice your concerns and questions with a provider you trust.

Pay special attention to how your provider talks about and addresses your weight. Red flags should go up when a provider tells you not to gain any weight at all, treats your size as something annoying, tells you that you should have lost weight before getting pregnant, or immediately assume you will have a difficult and complicated pregnancy just because you weigh more than what is thought of as the average woman. Any provider who makes you feel bad about yourself is not someone who is going to help you have a positive experience.

"If you have a weight Nazi doctor start to go off on you about your size, stand up and walk out of the office and don't look back. YOU are paying THEM, so doctors actually work for you, and as a paying customer, you don't have to take any crap from them, nor should you."—DeAnn R.

Developing a Good Patient-Provider Relationship

You and your provider must work as a team. Your provider gives you information, choices, and health care. You make informed decisions, express your needs, and ask questions. A good relationship means you have mutual respect for each other. Your provider must talk to you as if you are a thinking, feeling, reasonable, intelligent, and important person. She must give you choices, not orders. The health-care provider must also talk to you about things that might make you uncomfortable or worried, as long as it's done in a way that is supportive and not accusatory.

In return, you must treat your health-care provider with similar respect. Be receptive to suggestions or advice. Be honest with your health-care provider. Take recommendations seriously, and ask thoughtful questions. Think of yourselves as partners in your pregnancy. Being partners means you're on equal footing. Your health-care provider might be the expert in medical care, but you're the expert when it comes to your body and your comfort levels.

"My doctor was great. I was really nervous the first appointment. She said she had delivered healthy babies from women that were bigger than me and expected everything would go perfectly. She even said at one point that larger women 'do' pregnancy better—their balance isn't as affected, and they don't have the same weight-gain issues."—Margie P.

"Until something comes up, I believe you should be treated like any other pregnant woman. I know my OB did. He knows I know I am big, and I know he knows I am big. I asked the questions I needed to know about being big and pregnant."—Jennifer H.

"Both my providers treated me with respect and did not focus on my weight. When an issue with my weight was discussed, I never felt berated or shamed. I was very fortunate because I have heard horror stories."—Andrea H.

"Be honest, and ask for help if you need it. Doctors are there to assist you, not to judge you."—Sharon L.

"I am meeting with my OB and a perinatologist tomorrow. I am a potential high risk due to my weight, my age—thirty-seven—and the fact that I'm carrying twins. I will very quickly tell them that because I'm fat, it's important to me to work closely with my doctor and find a good nutritionist who is fat-positive and can help me have a healthy pregnancy without making me feel scared or worried."—Liz O.

"I had one OB who was super nice to me throughout the pregnancy. He was highly unusual. I can recall him saying I looked great whenever he saw me, which did make me feel a little better, and after the baby as I slimmed down, he praised me as well, but would say you looked great before, too, you know."—Michelle C.

"My midwife did not weigh me at all. She was great."—Rachel G.

"I said, 'Look, I'm not happy about my size, but I'm happy to be pregnant. How do I make the best of it?' My doctor was great. She said, 'Do NOT stress about your weight. Try to keep the weight gain minimal. Just enjoy the pregnancy.'"—Liz R.

"She told me that my weight might cause gestational diabetes or preeclampsia, but that we would cross that bridge IF we came to it. She basically told me to eat right for both of us, but never once made me feel like my weight was horrible or bad for the baby. If your doctor makes you feel bad about yourself, it is time to get a new doctor."—Becky A.

"My doctor was never concerned with my weight. I had smoked prior to pregnancy, and he told me that whenever I wanted to smoke, to eat something instead. He saw my weight gain as a positive sign that I wasn't smoking."—Vanessa R.

"I think it is very important to find a provider that is respectful of you and size friendly. Plus-size ladies can get pregnant and can have healthy babies! The medical community needs to recognize this."—Jennifer N.

"Be very up-front with your doctor about your concerns. You know you are overweight—so does your doctor. The two of you are working as a team to have a healthy pregnancy, for both you and the baby. Don't be embarrassed or ashamed—you are who you are, and you are now pregnant. Being overweight is a medical condition. If you only had one leg, would you be ashamed to mention it to your obstetrician? Of course not!"—Carla R.

Educate Yourself

Another important component to your relationship with your health-care provider is whether you are informed. Reading this book and other regular pregnancy books is an excellent way to arm yourself with information. It's hard to ask the right questions if you don't know what the possibilities and risks are. Once you are an informed patient, you can ask thoughtful questions that allow your provider to see that you have some basic knowledge about pregnancy and your condition, thus making him or her more comfortable giving you in-depth answers.

Some people have a tendency to hide from things that scare or worry them. Ignoring it won't make it go away. Take control of your health care. Learn all you can on your own, and ask questions of your provider.

"Be informed! Read books, gather information. Try to educate yourself as much as possible. It makes things a little less scary."—Jennifer N.

"I think I put my doctor's mind at ease at the first appointment when I asserted that I had done my research and knew I didn't need to gain much weight to sustain the baby through pregnancy. You will only help yourself if you walk in as the educated party on many subjects. A little research and a good pregnancy book will do the trick. There were very few times when the doctor surprised me, which meant I always had intelligent questions to ask that made me feel in control of my treatment."—Richelle H.

"The most helpful thing I did was be proactive! I educated myself very well on the effects of being pregnant and overweight. I would approach the doctor like I was the expert rather than he with comments and mutual dialogue rather than questions."—Dana C.

Dealing with Insensitivity

Although most providers will tell you that they would never want to make a patient feel uncomfortable or awkward, we're all human, and a provider or staff member might at some point say or do something that makes you feel hurt, embarrassed, or uncomfortable. Often these moments are caused not by intentional malice, but by insensitivity. If this happens, and you are comfortable doing so, speak up and say "What you just said hurt my feelings" or "When you say things like that, it makes me feel as if I do not have your complete respect." A good provider will apologize and make certain this never happens again. If you discover an ongoing pattern of this kind of behavior, you need to find a new health-care provider. Saying nothing means that the pattern of behavior will continue, and your self-esteem will probably suffer. You must remember that you deserve to be treated with kindness and respect at all times—it's not an extra benefit only accorded to thin women!

Life coach Ann Leach, coauthor of *Goal Sisters: Live the Life You Want with a Little Help from Your Friends*, recommends, "If your doctor is giving you negative feedback, I would take ten minutes of your appointment time to share your feelings with him/her. This professional is to be on your success team. Yes, they may be concerned about your weight on your pregnancy and life afterward—that is their job. Yet the way they communicate that is important. If you don't like their style, let them know, and ask for a change. You deserve it!"

"Some nurses acted like they didn't know why the blood-pressure cuff wasn't fitting. Is there really not that many pregnant heavy women? I used to think they did this on purpose."—Jennifer H.

"I had to see one of my OB's colleagues for one monthly visit during my first pregnancy. He was an older man. He shook his head and told me 'You're too fat. Don't gain much more weight.' I came out of the office near tears and felt six inches tall."—Cheryl H.

"I've found sadly that most doctors are not that helpful when it comes to discussing weight with their patients. My advice is this. If your doctor isn't supportive about your weight struggle—or even tries to make you feel badly about it—switch doctors if possible, or just nod and smile while they talk. Do not let anyone, especially your doctor, a person who makes their money off your condition, make you feel badly about your weight gain. This is a tough enough time. Pregnancy changes all kinds of things in your body, and to have to deal with a doctor who's not sympathetic is too much to add. I had a friend who was afraid to go into the exam room after stepping on the scale because she was afraid to suffer her doctor's wrath."—Michelle C.

"I was in a midwifery practice. In my seventh month of pregnancy, with no warning, they said I was too large to stay in that practice and shuttled me off to another one. I felt completely bushwhacked, like I'd failed a test I didn't even know I was taking! I was so angry. I called the head of the practice and let her have it—and she treated me from then on. I still think there is a lot of abuse and mistreatment of large women. I have no doubt about it."—Liz R.

"My nurse practitioner was less supportive. She recommended Weight Watchers (which refused to offer me a pregnancy plan). When I told her that they refused my business, she recommended Diet Cokes® and salads. I requested a different nurse at that point." —Vanessa R.

"With my first pregnancy I remember towards the end going in and my doctor telling me that I had gained nine pounds in one week and that I had better do something about that. What exactly I was supposed to do, I'm not sure. I do know that was one of the most embarrassing moments I've ever had. My husband was in there, too, which made it even worse. I almost canceled my appointment for the following week because I didn't want to go in and face her again. My third pregnancy with my twins I went to a different doctor who was slightly overweight herself, and she never made a comment about my weight gain, I think because she was someone who understood what it's like to struggle with your weight."—Beth U.

"I remember one doctor said something like 'With women your size, we can't really get an accurate reading on fundal height.' I don't think he was trying to be rude or judgmental, but his tone was offensive, and just those words made me feel like I wasn't receiving the same prenatal care as my thinner counterparts."—Dana C.

"For my second pregnancy, I switched from my doctor. I went to a woman who was highly recommended. The first appointment, she refused to even look for the heartbeat saying I was too big. Everything she discussed, she ended with 'I mean, you are X pounds!' I stayed with her through twenty weeks. After my second gestational diabetes test before twenty weeks (I had not had a problem with GD in my first pregnancy, but apparently my size alone convinced her that I needed testing) I went back to my own doctor."—Margie P.

"I've had Ob/Gyns make me feel terrible about the weight gain. I can recall during the first pregnancy, the group of doctors I saw was particularly harsh. They sat me down and made

me write down everything I was eating and then critiqued it. The woman said 'Peas? Why would you eat peas?' She chastised me for having bananas. They would threaten that if I didn't stop gaining weight, they'd have to repeat the glucose test, which had been nightmarish because the solution made me vomit and I had to drink it again. I refused to let them make me feel bad. I'll admit the first few times they put me through this, I cried on the way home. Then my uncle gave me a pep talk. The next time I went in, I just smiled the whole time, acted completely unbothered by the entire exchange. They did seem to let up somewhat, but the entire pregnancy was unpleasant because of their reaction."
—Michelle C.

"My doctor liked to make fun of my weight and made me feel uncomfortable. I changed doctors right away."—Ali S.

Dealing with Uncomfortable Moments

Even if you have a health-care provider you are comfortable with and who treats you with respect, you may have some uncomfortable moments relating to your body during the course of your pregnancy care. You might simply feel embarrassed at some point to have anyone see your naked body, or you might suddenly feel self-conscious about your size during an exam. It can also get tiring to always have your weight monitored, discussed, and tracked.

If you are working with a size-friendly health-care provider, he will not purposely do or say anything to cause you embarrassment or shame. Sometimes though, these feelings can just well up from within you. If you feel this way at any point, remind yourself that your health-care provider has seen hundreds of bodies of all different shapes and sizes. Yours is not anything new or different and doesn't cause her to bat an eye. You can also be certain that your health-care provider has seen larger bodies than yours.

Health-care providers have truly seen it all. You have nothing to feel embarrassed about. If you start to feel uncomfortable, remind yourself that he is not having any kind of reaction, and any feelings of shame or embarrassment are unfounded. Remind yourself that you are a beautiful and worthwhile woman, and while your pregnant body may be different from the one you are used to, or different from other pregnant bodies, it is definitely nothing to be embarrassed about.

If you really feel as if you are going to simply sink into the floor or die of shame, tell your provider! Say "I'm feeling a little self-conscious right now" or "I'm feeling uncomfortable about my body right now." She will be quick to assure you that you have nothing to feel badly about or may offer you some additional privacy, such as a sheet to drape over yourself. If your provider does not offer positive reinforcement, think about switching to someone else. If you are uncomfortable and don't think you want to stay with this practice, make a change.

Don't be afraid to offer suggestions to your provider about how you can be made to feel more comfortable. Many offices have suggestion boxes, and others have general e-mail addresses. Some women find that standing on the scale backwards so they can't see the numbers, or doing the weighing themselves helps them through awkward weigh-ins. Sometimes a staff member is insensitive and simply pointing this out to the doctor or midwife will resolve the problem. Remember that the key to a good relationship with your provider is trust. If you feel the office is using a blood-pressure cuff that is too small for you, speak up. If your gown is not comfortable, say something. If you can trust your health-care provider to be considerate and kind to you, then you truly have nothing of which to be afraid or ashamed.

Remember also that your health-care provider must monitor your weight throughout the pregnancy. All women are weighed at each visit. This is important because a sudden loss or sudden large increase in weight can indicate potential problems for both mother and baby. You may be uncomfortable with all the constant focus on weight, but it is a crucial part of your care. Let your health-care provider do her job while you focus on having a happy and healthy pregnancy.

4

Testing, Testing, 1-2-3:
Medical Care and Tests During Pregnancy

or something that women have been doing since the dawn of time, there are a lot of medical tests involved with pregnancy. In fact, it sometimes seems like pregnancy is one long test, especially since you begin your pregnancy with a home test. But the tests are important because they can identify problems and allow you to get treatment, or allow you to breathe a sigh of relief when you have normal results.

Most plus-size women will have normal pregnancies, and all the testing is just a precaution. This chapter is going to take a look at tests that might in some way be impacted by weight (either the test results are changed by weight, weight makes it harder to do the test, or different testing is recommended for larger women). The idea is to help you understand how things might be slightly different for you as a plus-size mom, so that you can feel comfortable managing the tests. Although this chapter talks about the ways weight is involved with tests, it's completely possible that you won't have any of these problems, so don't spend your time worrying about them or expecting any of it to happen to you. Inform yourself, and then continue to enjoy your pregnancy.

Heartbeats

The baby's heartbeat is heard in office visits using a handheld ultrasound device called a Doppler. The Doppler produces only sound and no image. It's always difficult to locate the heartbeat early in pregnancy, and your health-care provider may not be able to locate it on your first few prenatal visits. Don't be alarmed if the heartbeat can't be found with the Doppler in the first trimester. Larger women sometimes feel self-conscious about this and are sure it is because of their size. Understand that this can (and often does) happen to women of average size, as well. If your provider is concerned about not being able to find a heartbeat, he may order an ultrasound.

"At my first visit, the midwife couldn't find the heartbeat, but I wasn't worried since that had happened to my skinny pregnant sister six months before!"—Carla R.

"That first visit where they try to get the heartbeat is the worst. For both kids, I remember feeling like I should somehow suck my gut in or something. With my second, I remember the doctor telling me that it is very difficult to find the heartbeat that early in pregnancy."—Belinda Z.

"At twelve to thirteen weeks, she couldn't find [the heartbeat]. At fourteen, she usually could. It usually just meant an early ultrasound for me, which I never minded. I hated having my belly checked for the heartbeat because they had to burrow in my lower stomach to do so."—Margie P.

"First pregnancy, first time we had to go into the ultrasound room to hear the heartbeat. When he couldn't find it the first time, I panicked. My OB was quite calm and said it was probably due to my 'extra fluff.' After that, it would happen here and there, and I would not worry. I would say, 'Meet you in the ultrasound room.' We always got the information we needed and still got good pictures to take home."—Jennifer H.

"Both my pregnancies we were not able to hear the heartbeat via Doppler at my twelve-week appointment, at which time they did an ultrasound to confirm everything was OK, and then at my fifteen-week appointment, they heard the heartbeat without a problem."—Andrea H.

Ultrasounds

Ultrasounds provide an image of the baby on a computer screen and allow your care provider to check for abnormalities, the baby's sex (if you want to know it), and the baby's size and development. Research has shown that ultrasounds are not harmful to the baby, even if you have many of them during your pregnancy.

There are two kinds of ultrasounds. Transvaginal ultrasounds are usually done early in pregnancy when the baby is smaller, up to week fourteen of the pregnancy. A wand is inserted in the vagina, and the ultrasound is done through the cervix, rather from the outside of the abdomen. You'll need to remove your pants for this type of ultrasound, but will be given a sheet. Many health-care providers ask you to insert the wand yourself. It's not painful. The wand is then controlled from the outside by the technician. A transvaginal ultrasound is in no way affected by your weight, so there should be no worries about your size impacting the results. This type of ultrasound is very helpful in accurately dating the pregnancy, and if you have irregular periods (which is common among plus-size women), getting an ultrasound can be the only way to get an accurate date.

Transabdominal ultrasounds are done after week fourteen by moving a wand around the outside of the stomach. You'll need to lift up your shirt and roll down the waist of your pants for this. You may feel as though the technician is pressing extra hard to get a good exterior ultrasound image, but pressure is used for all ultrasounds, not just yours. There is a chance that a woman's size can have some impact on the quality of the ultrasound image because adipose (fat) tissue absorbs the ultrasound waves. The most recent ultrasound equipment has special high-resolution scanning probes and special settings for larger women that make the imaging more accurate. Note though that most health-care providers' in-office machines are not this current, so you might have a problem with this equipment. If the technician can't see everything he or she needs to, a second ultrasound done at a later date (when the baby's size or position has changed) or an ultrasound on a newer machine may be recommended.

There are some techniques during ultrasounds that have been found to improve the results for plus-size women. One is to ask the woman to lift up the lower part of her abdomen and have the probe placed underneath that area, just above the pubic bone. If you have a lot of scans, you'll get used to this, and some women just automatically do this when they lay down for an ultrasound. Don't be embarrassed. It's no different than the technician asking you to lift your leg or move your body to a different position on the table. Scanning near the bellybutton is also helpful. Both of these areas have relatively little fat tissue regardless of your size and can give technically good scans.

The second-trimester ultrasound (usually at sixteen to twenty weeks) is performed to detect any evidence of birth defects, search for "markers" indicative of chromosome problems, and confirm the dating of the pregnancy. Certain chromosome problems or spina bifida can be screened for by ultrasound. Although the ultrasound can't completely exclude these conditions 100 percent, if the ultrasound is normal, the likelihood or the risk that the baby has these conditions is low, don't panic. It does not necessarily mean your baby has one of these problems. At that point, your health-care provider may refer you to a specialist for a high-resolution ultrasound and consultation. Occasionally an amniocentesis may be recommended. If the ultrasound is inconclusive about these problems, then an amnio would be recommended. In plus-size women, the ultrasound may be performed a bit later (eighteen to twenty weeks) so that a better-quality image can be obtained. Ultrasounds may also be used to monitor the baby's growth during the pregnancy.

"The ultrasound technician at my doctor's office told me there was too much fat in the way to see the baby's sex. It was extremely upsetting for me as I had my heart set on finding out."—Julie M.

"I remember lying on the table for the ultrasound and just feeling so huge and awful. But I took a deep breath and reminded myself that the technician does this all day long and is used to pregnant bellies and women of all sizes."—Beth F.

"The only problem was getting a good view of the heart toward the end. They used the vaginal device and pushed it in my bellybutton to get a better view of the baby's heart, and it hurt really bad."—Deb P.

"I had trouble with ultrasounds. They had to push very hard."—Melissa S.

"The only thing that has irritated me about my doctor so far is that she has put off my ultrasound because she says that since I'm overweight, it'll be easier to see the baby if we do it later. But, on the other hand, I've heard that the longer you wait, the harder it is because the baby is too large to get the whole picture. I would have rather she left weight out of the issue and had her tell me 'because this is what I do.' I would definitely have preferred that answer to the one I got."—Jill G.

"We did have to have multiple anatomical ultrasounds to check on the baby's development. They weren't able to see all the things they wanted. They said this was because of fetal position and movement. I have a feeling my size could have contributed to it as well, but they never mentioned that aspect of it."—Jennifer N.

"I had a horrible experience with the doctor who read the ultrasound. My in-laws and husband were there with me, and the doctor came in before the ultrasound and said, 'I just want you to know we probably won't be able to tell the sex of the baby or even get any really good pictures since you are one of our thicker patients. Don't be disappointed.' I was horrified and embarrassed beyond belief. I cried all the way through the procedure. As it turned out, my size didn't affect anything. We found out the baby was a boy, and we got some great views of him, but the whole experience left me bitter."—Carla R.

Fundal Height

Throughout your pregnancy, your care provider will use a measuring tape to measure the size of your uterus (called fundal height) while you lie on your back. The height in centimeters usually corresponds to the week of pregnancy you are in. So, for example, if you measure 32 cm, your baby is the size of a thirty-two-week-old fetus. Your health-care provider presses and feels the top and bottom of the uterus, which can be located even if your abdomen is very thick. It is possible that your baby's size might be overestimated or that your health-care provider may have a difficult time feeling your uterus well enough, but if your provider is concerned about the baby's size, she may order an ultrasound to obtain a more accurate reading.

You shouldn't feel uncomfortable about having your stomach measured. Since it happens at each of your prenatal appointments, you'll probably get used to it. Remember that all pregnant women go through this, and it's a normal part of a prenatal visit. There's no need to undress, and most women just wiggle their pants down and lift up their shirt. If you feel uncomfortable during these visits, talk to your provider

"I hated getting my stomach out to have it measured. I always felt like a whale lying there. One doctor said to me that it is hard to get accurate measurement in larger women, and that made me feel embarrassed. With my second baby, they thought he was going to be much bigger than he was, and I think that my size had something to do with that."—Lee T.

"My first OB, who I saw until I was twenty-eight weeks, never even bothered to measure my fundal height. I knew they weren't doing it because of my weight. When I went to my new OB, she measured me, but didn't tell me the number and said, 'Well, I can't really rely on this number because so much of it is you, not the baby.' I was very embarrassed."—Jennifer

about your feelings, or switch to a provider who makes you feel more comfortable.

Other Screening Tests

Obese women may be at a slightly higher risk for certain types of birth defects such as spina bifida and congenital heart disease. Don't be overly concerned since in real terms the chance of this happening to you is not that high. To make sure everything is fine though, obese women are often encouraged to have a maternal-serum-alpha-fetoprotein (MSAFP) blood test done (see page 117 for a description of this test) as well as a high-resolution second-trimester ultrasound scan. The ultrasound should be performed by an experienced sonographer or a maternal-fetal medicine specialist and is used to detect birth defects such as open neural-tube defects (see page 99 for more information about this). Due to the increased risk of fetal heart defects, fetal echocardiography (an ultrasound of the fetal heart) should be done, usually between eighteen and twenty-two weeks. This test is usually performed by a maternal-fetal medicine specialist or pediatric cardiologist with a special interest in the fetal heart (fetal cardiology).

If your health-care provider recommends these screening tests, don't be alarmed. Remember he or she is there to make sure both you and your baby are and remain healthy, and this means being on the lookout for anything that could possibly affect you. For most women, the tests will show that absolutely nothing is wrong. You shouldn't be insulted if your health-care provider suggests additional screening tests because of your weight (although that can be hard to manage if you are treated in a disrespectful way). These tests are not invasive and will give you additional peace of mind that your baby is doing well. And the more ultrasounds you have, the more often you'll get to see your baby.

Amniocentesis

Amniocentesis is a procedure that allows your physician to remove and test a small portion of the amniotic fluid for abnormalities. An ultrasound is done at the same time so your doctor can see where the baby is and avoid harming it. A needle is then inserted through the abdominal wall, and a small portion of the amniotic fluid is withdrawn for testing.

This procedure is done to test for chromosome abnormalities (such as Down's syndrome) between fifteen and twenty weeks. It can also identify spina bifida. Amnios are important because there are some genetic disorders that can only be identified using an amnio. Amniocentesis is performed if MSAFP is elevated, the quad or triple screen shows an increased risk of chromosome problems, the ultrasound detects an abnormality, because the mother is older than thirty-five, or if both parents are carriers for genetic disorders like sickle cell anemia or cystic fibrosis (although these are more commonly tested for with blood work now). Being overweight alone is *not* a reason for an amnio.

Some women are concerned that their size will affect the procedure or that the doctor will not have a long enough needle. This is rarely the case. Special length needles with highly echogenic tips, which can be seen very easily by ultrasound, may be used for plus-size patients. You should remember that it's not the length of the needle, but its thickness that relates to discomfort. Amniocentesis needles are very thin to minimize discomfort. The standard description by physicians is that the procedure is not much more uncomfortable than having blood drawn, although each woman has a different experience.

Some women also worry that somehow their weight will make it difficult for the provider to accurately withdraw the fluid without harming the baby. Weight has no impact on the safety of the amnio. The ultrasound allows the doctor to accurately place the needle so the baby is not at risk.

If you need an amnio or your health-care provider recommends one, it is essential that you go to an experienced and skilled physician who is knowledgeable about the risks of the conditions being tested for and can offer options other than amniocentesis (such as a combination of blood tests and ultrasounds). The person performing the ultrasound should be highly trained and experienced in complex obstetrical ultrasound, and the physician performing the genetic amniocentesis should be experienced in doing them with plus-size women. This is generally a maternal-fetal medicine specialist (or perinatologist, a high-risk pregnancy specialist).

Nonstress Tests

A nonstress test is performed by placing a belt with a Doppler on it around your stomach to monitor the baby's heartbeat. These tests are normally done twice a week when they are needed. Size can make it more difficult to pick up a reading (just as with the handheld Doppler, fat or adipose tissue absorbs the Doppler ultrasound waves). The belt might have to be moved around or the monitors pressed against you by hand. If there is still difficulty with the test, an ultrasound biophysical assessment of the baby can be done. A biophysical profile looks at the baby's behavior (movement, muscle tone, and breathing motions) as well as the amniotic fluid. When this profile has normal results, it is very reassuring that the baby is doing well.

"They had trouble with the nonstress test to monitor the baby's heartbeat. They called the fat belly 'extra tissue.' It was embarrassing, but I was alone in a room, so only me and the nurse knew about it."—Peggy M.

5
Weighing the Facts:
The Truth About Plus-Size Pregnancy Weight Gain

Whether you're upset at the thought of gaining weight while pregnant or looking forward to a time in your life where some weight gain is expected, you need to know the facts about weight gain during pregnancy for plus-size women.

What the Experts Recommend

Obstetricians usually do not recommend that a plus-size woman go through a pregnancy without gaining weight. Weight gain is a necessary part of pregnancy for almost all women. How much weight is recommended can differ from doctor to doctor and with each patient's situation. In general, it is recommended that large-size women gain no more than fifteen to twenty pounds during pregnancy. This is in contrast to the twenty-five- to thirty-five-pound weight gain recommended for average-size women.

Most prenatal caregivers prefer to see patients gain weight slowly and gradually. A sudden increase in weight can signal problems such as preeclampsia. While slow weight gain is recommended, most women tend to gain more weight in the last two trimesters, so weight gain during these months tends to be faster than in the previous three months.

In some instances, a doctor may recommend a smaller weight gain if a woman is dangerously overweight or faces certain health concerns. It's important to consult your health-care provider and ask exactly how much weight he recommends for you. (See Chapter 6 for information about how to manage your weight gain.)

"I was very nervous about gaining weight since my doctor said I should only gain fifteen pounds total. I am pretty sure I gained about twenty-five to thirty pounds total. I stayed positive by eating foods I knew were good for the baby. He was my main concern. So even though I gained weight, I knew the foods I was eating were good for the baby."—Julie M.

"I have heard some doctors recommend that plus-size women don't gain ANY weight during pregnancy (luckily not mine). This is ridiculous! There is a baby growing inside you—of course you are going to gain weight!"—Jennifer N.

"As of now, I'm sixteen weeks and haven't gained a pound."—Melanie L.

"Being pregnant was the only time that I did not feel horrible for gaining weight."—Shannan E.

"I set out with my first pregnancy vowing that I was going to be so good and eat only healthy foods and gain no more than twenty-five pounds. In reality, I gained over sixty pounds. I was very self-conscious about it, especially at the weigh-ins at the doctor's office. I used to dread the weigh-ins more than any physical exam. But my baby was always doing fine, and I tried to keep positive by reminding myself that was the most-important thing."—Beth U.

"I only gained nine pounds the entire pregnancy. I was losing a pound here and there. Bigger women sometimes lose weight instead of gaining. The baby takes what it needs from us."—Deb P.

"I said with both pregnancies I was going to really try not to gain, but with both I gained around forty-five pounds. It did not bother me. I was having a baby. Plus, it made me look even-more pregnant."—Jennifer H.

"I had a goal—no more than twenty pounds of extra weight during the pregnancy. And I made it."—Liz R.

"All three pregnancies I gained nearly the same amount of weight. My OB told me that there was some research to support the idea that your body may have a set pregnancy weight gain. One pregnancy I carefully monitored what I ate. I walked routinely. I gained fifty pounds. The next pregnancy I was put on bed rest due to near-constant spotting. I was somewhat down and ate whatever I wanted. That included hot fudge sundaes. I gained fifty pounds. The third pregnancy I ate somewhere between the extreme 'eat whatever you want' and 'careful monitoring' and worked out religiously throughout the pregnancy. I gained fifty pounds."—Michelle C.

"I always gain about fifty pounds, no matter what. In the second trimester, I always gain about twelve pounds in six weeks, which can be disheartening, especially when the doctor gives you those looks. I didn't worry about gaining weight as much as I worried about the effects it was having on my health—bad back, swollen feet, heavy breathing, fatigue, etc. I knew I'd have to work really hard to lose the weight after pregnancy, but I also felt that a woman should never deny herself during pregnancy. Pregnancy, childbirth, and breastfeeding are a precious and brief time period, and I simply tell myself that the extra pounds were a testament to the vocation of motherhood."—Amelia M.

Being Realistic

Knowing the recommended guidelines for weight gain is one thing, but living with them is another. It can be just plain difficult to control weight gain while pregnant. Some women find they are always hungry. Other women find that eating is one of the best ways to control nausea. If you feel that you came into your pregnancy with a problem controlling weight gain, you'll probably find that it's not any easier to deal with while pregnant. Lots of things change during pregnancy, but pregnancy also triggers an automatic desire to nurture your growing child. Dealing with weight gain is one of the biggest issues plus-size women have with pregnancies. Gaining weight can feel completely natural while it's happening, but it's important to consider the big picture.

You need to decide how you're going to look at weight-gain issues during your pregnancy. You don't want to beat yourself up for every pound you gain, feel like the entire world is monitoring your weight gain, or focus your attention exclusively on your weight. It's easy to get yourself into a tailspin and go to one or the other extreme with this—refuse to care about weight you are gaining or get too upset about each ounce you put on. You do, however, want to take care of yourself and your baby. This means gaining some weight, but not letting yourself gain too much. If you gain twenty-five pounds instead of twenty, it's most certainly not the end of the world. If your doctor recommends a three-pound average gain each month and one month you come in and find you've gained five instead of three, you're not a bad person or a terrible mother.

Realize that weight gain during pregnancy can be a bit quirky. You may not gain any weight for a week or two and then suddenly put on two or three pounds in one week. It's important to focus on weight gain as a general concept. Try to stick to the goal your prenatal caregiver sets for you, but don't panic if you gain more in one week than you planned.

If you are horrified by weight gain during pregnancy (and this is common, particularly if you were a dieter before pregnancy), remind yourself that you gain weight for a reason. If you really feel like this is one time in your life when you want to let loose and eat as you please, consider the consequences carefully and try to let loose in small spurts.

"I was a patient in a midwifery practice, and they were wonderful to me. I told them at my very first visit how worried I was about how much I weighed and how that would affect me and the baby. They were very understanding and said that all three of them had seen many patients who were overweight have happy, healthy pregnancies. They told me that they would like to see me gain only between twenty-five and thirty-five pounds, but that they would not put me on a diet and that they knew my body would take care of the baby. They were right. Their confidence and positive attitude really helped me a lot. I stopped worrying about my weight gain when the midwife told me that I would gain just as much weight as the baby needed and that I should look at my changing body as a positive experience instead of a negative one. Your body will take care of the baby, so just let it do what it needs to do. Surrendering that obsession is the first of many surrenders that come with the territory in parenting."—Carla R.

"It can be hard at first, especially if you were like me and were on a diet prepregnancy. It almost feels like you are betraying yourself to allow yourself to gain weight, but you have to realize it is what nature intended. Try to eat healthy—realize everything that goes into your mouth can help your baby if you choose the right foods. Then the weight won't seem so bad since you know you are helping your baby grow."—Jennifer N.

"I didn't gain a lot of weight during either of my pregnancies, but I remained philosophical about the whole process because I knew there was nothing I could do to stop it."—Sharon L.

What This Means for You

You should *not* try to go through your pregnancy without gaining any weight. Some women (and even some misinformed doctors) believe that it's best to go through a pregnancy without gaining a pound. Some people think that this will allow you to end up weighing less after the birth than before the pregnancy. Most health-care providers agree that no weight gain during pregnancy is unhealthy. A study in the *American Journal of Epidemiology* in 2003 showed a relationship between dieting or fasting early in pregnancy and an increased risk of neural-tube defects, so this should be a clear sign to you that you must eat. On the other hand, many women experience nausea or vomiting with no weight gain or weight loss during early pregnancy. This kind of weight loss does not increase the risk of birth defects, so don't worry if it happens to you.

Your body is not only growing a baby that is going to weigh about seven pounds, but you're also adding blood, amniotic fluid and a placenta. (See Chapter 2 for a breakdown of how much all of this weighs.) If you don't gain weight to do this, your body will drain its fat supplies, in essence putting your body on a diet while trying to support a new life. Andrea Henderson, birth doula (a doula is a trained birth assistant who works closely with the mother and focuses on encouraging and supporting her; unlike a midwife, most doulas do not actually deliver the baby), says, "I've often heard doctors chastising women for weight gain, limiting weight gain to ten to fifteen pounds, which is actually asking women to LOSE weight during pregnancy because the baby, placenta, fluids, blood volume, breast tissue, etc., weigh more than that alone! On the other hand, it is not uncommon for larger women to not gain or even lose weight during pregnancy—even if they are eating well."

Failing to gain enough weight during pregnancy can result in a low-birth-weight baby (under five-and-a-half pounds) who is at greater risk of developmental and health problems. It is, however, possible to be a plus-size mom and not gain any weight during pregnancy, but it is difficult to do and not always advisable. If your goal is to not gain any weight at all, first discuss this with your health-care provider. Next, see a nutritionist so that you can be certain the foods you are eating are providing everything your body and the baby's body need. Then, try to follow your plan, but don't starve yourself or fast.

A lot of the weight gain in the first half of pregnancy is fat or adipose tissue. If you begin pregnancy with large fat or adipose stores, you generally don't have to gain as much weight during pregnancy to assure a good outcome. Many plus-size women become concerned when they don't gain as much weight as their thinner counterparts during pregnancy, but this is usually not something to worry about. One way for your health-care provider to tell if your body is not getting enough nutrition is to check your urine for ketones. Ketones are a group of chemicals produced in the body when fat stores are broken down. They are then excreted in the urine and can be detected by chemical strips dipped in the urine. The urine dipsticks used routinely at each prenatal visit detectprotein, blood, sugar (glucose), and ketones. Pregnant women will frequently have ketones in their urine if they skip meals, so you should not worry if this happens occasionally. Ketones are also frequently seen in the first trimester when many women have nausea and vomiting and lose weight. Later in the pregnancy, however, ketones should not be consistently present in the urine. If you have not gained much weight during pregnancy, you should ask your health-care provider if you have ketones present in your urine at most of your prenatal visits. This would be an indication that you need to increase your caloric intake. On the other hand, if you are not gaining much weight, but you do not have persistent ketones in your urine, and the baby is growing well, it is probably an indication that all is well. Many plus-size women may gain little or no weight during the pregnancy and still have a healthy normal-sized baby.

You'll probably find that it's practically and emotionally difficult to prevent some weight gain during pregnancy. You are growing and nurturing a child inside your body, and part of your natural impulse is to feed and nourish that child. Many women feel strong impulses to eat lots of healthy foods, to respond to cravings, and to gain weight to help the fetus grow. These are natural pregnancy impulses, and it is OK to listen and respond to them. Your doctor or midwife will probably tell you, however, that it's not OK to view pregnancy as a time when you can eat whatever you want and gain as much weight as you want without consequences. You want to find a way to respond to your natural needs and urges without gaining too much weight. (See Chapter 6 for information about controlling appetites and urges while still feeling good about yourself and your pregnancy.) "The main thing to remember," says Leanne Ely, certified nutritional consultant and author of *Saving Dinner*, "is that you have to face your body postpregnancy. Eat smart, and eat healthy."

"Make sure your doctor knows that you're not sitting around eating bonbons all day—that you're eating your fruits and vegetables."—Amelia M.

Why Limiting Weight Gain is Important

While gaining weight is an important part of pregnancy, too much weight gain can create problems and unnecessary risks for you and your baby. Gaining more than the recommended amount can result in an overweight baby (more than nine pounds). A large baby can make a vaginal birth difficult or impossible, necessitating a C-section, with its intrinsic risks. A large baby is also at a higher risk for shoulder dystocia and birth trauma. (See Chapter 16 for more information about large-for-gestational-age babies.) A mother who gains too much weight during pregnancy increases her risk of hypertension, preeclampsia, and gestational diabetes. These are risks shared by any woman who gains too much weight during pregnancy—not just plus-size women.

Gaining too much weight can also result in more pregnancy-related discomfort such as groin muscle pain, ligament pain, back pain, and sore feet. And of course, gaining too much weight simply makes it harder to return to a prepregnancy weight after the baby is born. If you are short, your risks for all of these problems are higher than for other large women, so your doctor or midwife may recommend you gain even less weight than other plus-size women. If you believe you are shorter than most women, ask your provider about this.

Getting Past Weight

While weight gain is something your health-care provider will monitor and discuss with you, your entire pregnancy does not have to be, and should not be, about weight gain. Gaining some weight—but not a lot more than recommended—is certainly important, but it shouldn't be something that dominates your entire pregnant mind.

Many women find that they are better able to cope with weight gain, control it, and feel good about it during pregnancy because it's all linked to an important and magical outcome—a wonderful, healthy baby. When you think about gaining or controlling weight during your pregnancy, do so with your baby in mind. If you're disturbed by your weight gain, visualize where all of it is going. Close your eyes, and imagine your baby growing, your uterus expanding, and your blood volume increasing with each ounce.

If you find you are having a difficult time limiting yourself to the recommended weight gain, focus on the healthy baby you want to have. Remind yourself that this is what the entire process is about. You know you would do simply anything for this unborn child of yours, so try to keep that in mind when you are making daily food choices. There is nothing easy about controlling weight gain during pregnancy, though many health-care providers can certainly make it seem that way (especially the thin ones). They dispense the same advice to women every day and sometimes recite the information as if by rote, without really considering what they are asking of you. Acknowledge to yourself that controlling weight gain during pregnancy is a difficult mission, but one that you are willing to tackle for the benefit of your child.

"Weight gain during my first pregnancy bothered me. I was so worried it would be impossible to lose."—Beth U.

"One of the nurses exclaimed, 'Oh my God, WHAT are you eating?' To which I said, 'Food.' Then the doctor said I COULD develop toxemia, and my blood pressure COULD go up, and my baby COULD die. All of which I knew was overexaggeration. He said, 'Three meals a day. That's it.' I said, 'That's what I've been doing.' And he shook his head. I've found that ignoring it all is the best thing to do."—Amelia M.

"[Weight] was my biggest concern during the pregnancy. When I found out I was pregnant, one of my first thoughts was 'Oh no! I was supposed to lose weight before this happened!'

Fortunately, my midwife was very supportive and helped me by telling me that many women my size and larger had healthy pregnancies and deliveries."—Carla R.

"My doctor was very supportive. He explained to me that fat stored during pregnancy was normal, to provide breast milk for babies and that once I gave birth and started nursing, my weight would melt off. He said that every body reacts differently to pregnancy as far as weight gain. He made me feel secure and happy, so I wasn't worried about weight gain and stressed out instead of calm and focused on making a healthy baby."—Vanessa R.

"I was disappointed that I wasn't at my 'ideal' weight when I got pregnant the first time, but I really just concentrated on doing the best with eating and taking care of myself so I wouldn't jeopardize the health of the baby. I realized that my size wasn't as important as that."—Lisa B.

6

Staying Healthy

*S*taying healthy is probably at the top of your list right now. Every mother wants to create a healthy environment for her baby, but it's easy to worry about whether you're doing the right things and whether your weight is going to affect the baby. The best way to ensure a healthy baby is to have a healthy mom. Sometimes, when you're overweight, you can feel so bad about yourself that it's easy to allow yourself to treat your body poorly because after all, you think "I'm already fat, so why does it matter?" It *does* matter, and paying attention to diet and exercise during pregnancy will not only keep you feeling good, but will also help you avoid problems such as gestational diabetes.

This doesn't mean that you should turn your life upside down, work out until you faint, or subsist only on carrots and milk. It does mean that focusing on your health should be important to you and that it doesn't have to be a miserable experience. When you're used to being overweight, it's easy to think of healthy living as being burdensome or impossible. It really doesn't have to be, and if you can maintain your current level of health or slightly improve some things, it will go far toward your goal of a healthy pregnancy.

It's essential that you get solid nutritional information, either from your health-care provider or by seeing a nutritionist. It's equally important to discuss any exercise plans with your health-care provider. For most women, eating a reasonable diet and getting a decent amount of exercise isn't a problem, and your health-care provider will green light your plans. But it's always a good idea to have that conversation before making any major life changes.

"I was so scared when I found out I was pregnant that I would be unable to have my baby. I just want to tell people it can be done, and you can stay healthy as well. Don't let people get you down."—Julie M.

You Can Be Overweight and Healthy

There is this perception in our society that if you're overweight, you are a complete potato-chip-eating, candy-stuffing slug who never moves out of the recliner. You already know that's not true, and most overweight women do stay active. It's important to remember that while health and weight are linked in an important way, you can be larger than average and still be an active, healthy woman. You shouldn't assume, or let other people make you feel that just because you weigh a bit more, you aren't interested in health or you don't take care of yourself.

When you read about pregnancy risks and weight in media reports, you may come across information about things such as neural-tube defects and the conclusion that larger women are at a higher risk because of their diet. (See Chapter 7 for information.) Some material even goes so far as to suggest that plus-size women are nutritionally deficient (some reports have described overweight women as actually starving themselves of important nutrients)—as if they eat nothing other than bonbons, and salad or fruit never crosses their lips. Most of the women surveyed for this book said that they eat an appropriate amount of nutritionally sound foods and believe they are overweight because they either eat too much of everything (good foods included) or because they eat "bad" foods in addition to the good foods. No one who was interviewed said they subsist only on Twinkies, despite what the media might have us believe.

The basic key to being healthy is eating a nutritionally sound diet and getting moderate exercise—ideally, thirty minutes a day. If you're frightened by how this sounds, remember that a nutritionally sound diet doesn't mean eating plain chicken breasts and steamed broccoli all the time, and exercise doesn't mean running around a track until you can't breathe or putting yourself through an excruciating spinning class. Make sure your diet contains the appropriate amount from each food group, take your prenatal vitamin, and get enough calcium and protein. (See a nutritionist if you aren't sure about what exactly you should eat.) Walk, swim, lift small hand weights, or ride a bike to get exercise, and don't go at breakneck speed. Staying healthy while pregnant is an act of love for your child and shouldn't be torture.

It's also important to remember that even the healthiest people fall off the wagon sometimes. We all have our moments, and if you can't find time to take a walk for a few days, don't beat yourself up. If you have to have a big slice of cheesecake with chocolate sauce followed by a handful of peanut M&Ms, you haven't permanently sabotaged anything or done anything horrific. Be patient and tolerant with yourself.

"You can have a healthy pregnancy and be overweight at the same time. I'm living proof of that. I've done it three times. I believe you can be overweight, pregnant, and healthier than the general population. In fact when I take my thirty-minute walk at the YMCA, I zoom by many thin young men and women—and I'm eight months pregnant. My blood pressure is normal; my blood sugar levels are normal—I'm just bigger."—Dana C.

Dealing with Cravings and Appetite Changes

Because your body is changing, the foods you like and are interested in are going to change as well. We've all heard the stories about pickles and ice cream, but you never really know what you might end up craving. Some experts believe cravings are your body's way of asking for certain nutrients, so when a craving has some nutritional value, they recommend listening to it. Cravings for unhealthy foods don't have to be off-limits, though. *Everything in moderation* is a good motto to follow when pregnant. There's no evidence that larger women have worse or different cravings than any other women, so don't feel self-conscious about them.

Merry Rose, a certified nutritionist and owner of Rose Nutrition Center (*www.rosenutrition.com*), says, "If your cravings are for sugar, try satisfying them with sweet fruits like apples, berries, and melons. For fatty food cravings, make sure you are getting enough good fats in your diet, such as olive oil. Snacking on something with protein like vegetable sticks and hummus or a nut butter can satisfy cravings for fat."

If you find that you are repulsed by certain foods, avoid them. If you find that you just can't eat foods like milk or most proteins, talk to your health-care provider to make sure you're getting enough nutrients in your diet.

"One night I had to have cold Pepsi, but it had to be in a plastic bottle, not a can. Then there was the pizza-with-ground-beef-on-top stage. In one pregnancy, I could not eat any cooked vegetables (only raw) and in another I could not eat any chicken."—Brenda Z.

"Give in to your cravings sometimes. If you don't, you may find yourself bingeing one day."—Ali S.

"Cravings, yeah, you have them. Watch the rest of your diet the rest of the day, but when that craving hits, give in. The reason? If you don't eat what you want, you'll get frustrated, bitchy, annoyed, and want to eat everything else to try and satisfy the craving. Instead, just have it and get it out of your system."—Lisa B.

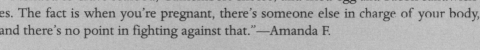

"I tended to crave seafood, Camembert cheese, and fried-egg-and-bacon sandwiches. The fact is when you're pregnant, there's someone else in charge of your body, and there's no point in fighting against that."—Amanda F.

"I need an avocado right now."—Lee T.

Dealing with Hunger

Especially at the beginning of your pregnancy, you may have very little appetite, but as your pregnancy progresses, you may find that you're hungry all the time. This can be a problem, especially if your health provider has limited your weight gain. You're caught between two conflicting desires. On one hand, you want to have a healthy pregnancy, not gain a lot of weight, and do what your health-care provider suggests. On the other, you have these very real and pressing physical needs to eat—like your body is just crying out for you to feed your baby. So how do you balance the two?

When you're hungry, you should eat, but if you can monitor the types and amounts of foods you eat, you will go a long way towards controlling weight gain. Instead of having a whole peanut-butter-and-pesto sandwich, take one piece of bread, and make half a sandwich, or just make it open face, so it feels like a full size. Tell yourself that if you want more when you've finished it, you can have it then. Try substituting healthier things for bad foods. Instead of having a candy bar, eat a cup of fat-free pudding. Eating small amounts more often will keep you from getting hungry enough to sit down and eat a whole pizza.

One woman interviewed for this book used apples to control her hunger. Whenever she was hungry, but believed she really didn't need to eat a lot, she would eat an apple. She would tell herself that once she had eaten the apple, if she still wanted the food she craved, she could have it. Most of the time, the apple satisfied her hunger, and she didn't need to eat whatever it was that was tempting her.

Sometimes thirst can be mistaken by your body for hunger. If you find you are desperately hungry, but are trying not to eat as much, have a large glass of water and see if that helps you feel full.

Dealing with hunger and appetite throughout pregnancy is definitely a struggle for many plus-size women. Perhaps the best way to deal with it is to first gather information (see later in this chapter) about how much you should be eating. Next, make every effort to eat the right foods in the right amounts. Finally, forgive yourself for falling off the wagon once in a while. This is not the same as giving yourself carte blanche to eat whatever you want during pregnancy. The key is to find a happy medium where you can eat healthily, control your calories, and still satisfy your body's needs.

"The best thing to remember is that you ARE eating for two, but one of you is teeny tiny. You really only need an extra 300 calories a day. Before you eat something, ask yourself if it was something you would want your baby eating, because essentially he will be eating it, too."—Vanessa R.

Eating a Healthy Diet

Most women have a good idea about which foods are healthy and which aren't, but pregnancy is a good time to brush up. Read a few pregnancy nutrition books (see Appendix), or consider seeing a nutritionist if you think you need some guidance. Eating right doesn't mean emptying the cupboards and restocking with tofu and lentils. It means making small adjustments in your diet to maximize what you're eating.

Nutritionist Merry Rose says, "The best diet for any pregnant woman is one consisting of whole, fresh food. This means eating whole grains instead of refined. As much as possible, eliminate from your diet caffeine, sugar, hydrogenated or partially hydrogenated oils and fats such as those found in margarine. Read labels. Entirely eliminate alcohol. Eat lots of fresh vegetables and fruits. Eat organic meat, poultry, and dairy products. Calcium intake should be about 1,200 mg per day.

Any pregnant woman, and plus-size women in particular, need to eat the most nutrient-dense food they can. Nutrient-dense food simply means foods that have the most nutrients for the least calories. Every time you eat something that is of low nutritional value, you are adding empty calories to your diet."

Protein is another essential element of your diet and you should get 60 grams per day. High protein diets are potentially harmful during pregnancy, so always discuss any diet or out of the ordinary food plan with your health-care provider.

Increasing Calories

If your health-care provider has given you the green light, you'll probably slightly increase your calorie intake during pregnancy in order to gain the recommended amount of weight. The usual recommendation is to increase calories between 100 and 300 per day, and normally this would slowly build throughout the pregnancy—needing closer to 100 calories in the first trimester and 300 in the third. It's important to really understand what these calories mean. An extra 100 calories is one banana. Three hundred is a chicken sandwich or crackers and cheese. It's not like adding another whole meal to your day.

The problem a lot of plus-size women face is how to gain the recommended amount of weight without gaining too much and how to increase calories without letting your eating get out of control. It's a fine line to walk for. The best way to get a grip on how much to eat is to see a nutritionist. If you can't afford to do this, at the very least, it's worthwhile to educate yourself about the calorie content of your diet. Learn how many calories you eat when not pregnant, and then see what the additional 300 calories recommended for pregnant women really means in terms of food you eat. Is it the same as a regular afternoon snack you normally have? Compare it to real food you usually eat so you can get a good sense of what it means in your life.

Eating Several Smaller Meals

In several places throughout this book (and in many other pregnancy books, as well), you'll find advice telling you to eat several small meals during the day to help deal with nausea and for other reasons. This sounds simple, but how do you really do it in practice? Does this mean you can't eat meals with your family? Does it mean you're going to have to interrupt your day for meal preparation every few hours? The easiest way to think of this is to plan on eating meals at regular times, but to eat a bit less than you normally would. So instead of having a bagel and fruit for breakfast, just have the bagel. Then add in two to three small snacks a day, but make sure the snacks are good food. Eating fruit, yogurt, or crackers with peanut butter is what you want to do, instead of eating chips or a candy bar. At dinner, don't have a second helping of spaghetti, knowing that you will need to eat something small later in the evening before you go to bed. You'll find that once you start eating this many meals a day, you are able to spread out your normal calorie intake across them.

Exercising

The American College of Obstetricians and Gynecologists (ACOG) says that a woman who was exercising before pregnancy can continue her prepregnancy routine with some changes. So if you liked to walk or swim before pregnancy, you should continue to do that. A 1997 report from the *American Journal of Epidemiology* showed that moderate amounts of exercise reduces the rate of gestational diabetes for overweight women, so exercise is an important way to stay healthy throughout your pregnancy.

Tips for Healthy Exercise

It's important to stay cool and well hydrated while exercising because extreme overheating can be dangerous for the baby. Some women read that and think they shouldn't do anything that will make them sweat. That's not the case at all. If the temperature under your arm is more than 101 degrees after exercising, then you're getting too hot. You can sweat and exert yourself without getting to that point. If you find you're having hot and cold flashes or have clammy hands, you should stop exercising and talk to your doctor. Staying hydrated (drinking water) while exercising will help keep your body temperature down, so be sure to have water with you.

After the first trimester, you should avoid exercising on your back because this can decrease blood flow to the baby. During the second and third trimesters, be aware of your shifting center of gravity, and avoid exercise that could cause a loss of balance. It's also a good idea to avoid exercise that could cause impact that could hurt the baby—no diving to get the volleyball or jumping on the trampoline. Also, during these later semesters, there is an increase in relaxin, which allows the joints and connective tissue to loosen, so it's important to avoid overstretching.

The March of Dimes, in a report called *Weight Matters,* recommends that overweight women continue being active during pregnancy, but avoid activities that create extreme fatigue. Exercise, but don't go crazy is the message.

Lisa Stone, ACE (a certification from the American Council on Exercise), creator of the DVD *Fit for 2 Step Aerobic Workout for Pregnancy* (*www.fitfor2.com*), recommends the following exercise program for larger women who aren't completely new to being active. "Walk for twenty to thirty minutes at a moderate pace three to five times a week, swim twenty minutes at a moderate pace three to five times per week, or do a combination of the two." Stone says that you should be able to talk through your workout. Breathing heavy and sweating are OK, but breathlessness is not. "Listen to your body! It will tell you when you've had enough. If something hurts or just doesn't feel right, don't do it. The pain is your body's way of telling you to stop."

If You're New to Exercise

If you didn't exercise before pregnancy, you can add some exercise to your life gradually if your doctor says it's OK. The key here is the word "gradually." If you didn't exercise before you got pregnant, it's too much to expect yourself to jump into a routine where you're huffing your way around the block for thirty minutes a day. Walk for five minutes today. Do it ten minutes tomorrow. If it hurts or if you're tired, stop and try again later. This is not about killing yourself. Start slowly, and remind yourself that every little bit you do helps your body and your baby. You also shouldn't feel like you've got to block out thirty minutes in one slot each day. You can do ten minutes of some kind of exercise three times a day if you want, once you work up to it.

Stone says, "For those pregnant women who are new to exercise, walking and swimming are two great places to start. Both are gentle on your joints and will allow you to increase the intensity. Pregnancy is a great time to learn to tune in to your body's signals during exercise. This is not a time to work through pain or discomfort." Lifting small weights (three pounds and lighter) is another great way to move your body without going overboard. Learn to do some basic arm exercises with these weights—you can even do them while watching TV.

Rochelle Rice, author of *Real Fitness for Real Women: A Unique Workout Program for the Plus-Size Woman* (*www.RochelleRice.com*), recommends gentle stretching exercises. "Focus on abdominal exercises. Sit in a chair and draw your navel and abdominal muscles in and up. Hold it for a count of ten, and try to increase the number of times. You can do this anywhere, while driving in a car or watching TV. This will improve abdominal muscles and strengthen the back." Rice also says plus-size pregnant women need to focus on alignment. "The plus-size body is very good at adapting to weight. Now you're adding a baby to it, and you want to stay aligned. Make sure your head is on top of your spine and not craning toward a computer screen. Focus on upper-back muscles to help support the extra weight of breasts during pregnancy."

To improve alignment, she suggests sitting exercises. Make sure you can feel the chair through the bones in your butt or your glutes and are sitting on it completely evenly. Sit totally aligned. Another exercise is to sit on the floor with legs forward and heels on the ground. Bend toes down to the floor and up. This will prevent shin splints if you walk for exercise, which a lot of plus-size women do. Another is to sit on the floor with legs out in front, making sure your thighbones are aligned. They tend to turn out in plus-size women. She also recommends that if you walk for exercise, pay attention to the noise of your feet on the ground. "It should sound like 'step, step, step, step,' but if you hear 'step, bang, step, bang,' then you know you're not walking in alignment and one foot is hitting the floor harder. Pay attention to walking evenly and you will feel better."

Stone recommends loose, breathable clothing, like a loose T-shirt with bike shorts or yoga pants. "The most important articles of clothing are a well-fitting, supportive bra and well-fitting, shoes," she points out. Rice says, "Plus-size women tend to wear heavier clothing to cover themselves up. Dress in fewer lightweight clothes when you exercise." Rice also recommends exercising in a well-ventilated area so you can stay cool.

Additionally, Stone recognizes that many women avoid exercise during pregnancy because they simply aren't feeling well in general. "In many cases exercise reduces many of the negative side effects of pregnancy, such as nausea and fatigue. So if there is any way they can force themselves to at least try to move their bodies, maybe they'll feel better.

That said, for those women who are so nauseous that they're vomiting on a daily basis, they may need to forgo exercise until that nausea passes completely."

The thought of an "exercise program" might sound a little overwhelming, so instead, just think of it this way. Try to find time on most days to move your body, whether it means taking a walk around the block or mall or splashing in the pool. You don't have to join a gym and buy expensive workout clothes. Sometimes plus-size women get caught up in the idea that they aren't athletic or don't know how to "exercise." Stop thinking of it as something so formal and frightening. Just resolve to do something every day that gets you moving. If it hurts, stop. You're not trying to win a marathon, you're just trying to move around and stay healthy.

"Walk, even if you go to the mall and walk around to the different stores."—Jennifer W.

"Yoga, it does wonders for my back."—Angelique G.

"To be honest, I was so scared to exercise for fear of losing the baby. I didn't have any real reasons for this fear. I just knew being my size and pregnant was already a risk, so I stopped."—Julie M.

"I liked the elliptical machine—low impact, adjustable resistance."—Vanessa R.

"Walking was really great for me. I also got a prenatal yoga tape that I loved."—Becky A.

"I joined a pregnancy exercise class. It was just once a week and very gentle exercise, but fun and just a nice thing to do."—Amanda F.

"I was told I had to quit aerobics at the gym because my body got too hot and I would miscarry. So I took short walks a couple times a day and tried to be gentle with myself."—DeAnn R.

"Back when I was a size 14, I never exercised. But it seems to me that as my body has gotten older (and bigger) that exercise is just an essential component in feeling good for me, and that was true during pregnancy, too. I don't do it to get thin, I do it to stay healthy."—Lee T.

"Swimming and walking were the two things I enjoyed doing while pregnant. Both are easy for someone who is already overweight to do without becoming too tired."—Beth U.

7

Does My Weight Affect My Pregnancy?

*E*very woman faces some kind of risk in pregnancy. For example, babies born to women older than thirty-five are at a higher risk for Down's syndrome, and those born to parents of Jewish descent are at a higher risk of Tay-Sachs disease, but most pregnancies have a happy ending. No one is guaranteed a perfect pregnancy or a perfect baby, but this doesn't mean you can't deliver a healthy baby, stay healthy, and feel good about yourself while being plus-size. Most babies *are* healthy, and *most* pregnancies are normal. So yours very likely will be, too.

Health-care providers deal with all kinds of risks in pregnancy and are usually able to manage them to successful outcomes. While it's true that being overweight can impact the risk for certain conditions or problems, this doesn't mean any of these will happen to you or even that they are likely to happen to you. Keep in mind that there are lots of things worse than being overweight and pregnant. Since half of the general population is overweight, plus-size moms have healthy pregnancies all the time.

Although you are most likely going to have a happy and healthy pregnancy, it's important to understand your potential risk factors. This chapter will lay out the facts, not scare you or make you feel guilty. You can choose to read about the potential problems and concerns now and then let yourself move past them and have a relaxed pregnancy, or you might even decide there's no reason to read this chapter unless a problem comes up in your pregnancy and you need information. Gather the information you need, but don't let it scare you, upset you, or depress you. Return to this chapter if your health-care provider has concerns about any particular conditions. Remember, you are likely to remain healthy and have a baby that's healthy, too.

Understanding Risk

It's essential to remember when reading about the risk of health problems that a risk is just that—only a chance or probability. You are not guaranteed to develop or face any of the problems discussed in this chapter. In fact, it's more likely that you won't be faced with them since the risk for each is reasonably small. It's important, however, to be educated so you can ask your doctor informed questions, understand anything out of the ordinary that may come up, and rest comfortably, knowing the facts. Your health-care provider is trained to look at and think about risk factors—and that's what you want him or her to do. You want someone who is experienced and knowledgeable to be on the lookout for any potential problems. Let your health-care provider weigh these risks for you, and remind yourself that this is preventive care.

In recent years, there has been a lot in the news about the link between being overweight and certain pregnancy problems, but the stories contain very little information explaining how small the risks really are, so that many women feel overwhelmed and frightened. While we all know that every time we get in a car, there's a risk of getting into an accident, this doesn't deter us from getting in the car and going to work or to the store. There is risk in almost everything we do every day. If we spent all our time obsessing about our risk factors, none of us would be very functional. What we can do is find out how to minimize our risk (like wearing a seat belt in a car or taking a prenatal vitamin while pregnant). With pregnancy that means educating yourself and talking to a doctor or midwife and following his or her advice.

As you read this chapter keep in mind what percentages really mean. If there is a 4-percent risk of an occurrence, that means that out of every 100 women, only four will develop or have to deal with it—and out of 1,000 women, only 40 will encounter it. Converting statistics into real terms can help you think rationally about them.

Another very important point to keep in mind when reading about risks is that many studies link the mother's weight with conditions or outcome, yet do not separate out the women with gestational diabetes. (See the section about gestational diabetes later in this chapter.) Women with gestational diabetes are at a higher risk for almost every condition and outcome discussed. If you don't have gestational diabetes, this means your risk may not be as high as the studies indicate. If you do have gestational diabetes, it means you should work with your health-care provider to keep your condition under control.

Don't be overwhelmed by statistics. For some conditions, you'll see that larger-size women have a risk that is two or three times greater than that of average-weight women. This sounds scary until you realize how low the risk is for average-weight women. Something that is a 1-percent risk among all pregnant women and has twice the risk in larger women puts your risk at only 2 percent, or two out of 100. Having a double or triple risk factor then doesn't seem as frightening.

It's also important to know that with some conditions, family history can play a critical role in increasing your risk. Be sure to talk to your doctor or midwife about occurrences in your family and consider genetic counseling if it is recommended.

Understanding Terms

Medical studies that assess the impact of the mother's weight on pregnancy and on the baby use specific medical terms to define certain groups of women. Unfortunately, some of these terms are less than flattering. But you need to understand them if you're going to make sense of the medical findings.

First, you need to understand the term BMI (body mass index). Body mass index compares weight and height and outputs a two-digit number. Calculate your prepregnancy BMI at the National Institutes of Health Web site at *http://nhlbisupport.com/bmi/*, or use the chart available at *http://www.nhlbi.nih.gov/guidelines/obesity/bmi_tbl.htm*. You can also calculate your BMI using this formula:

$$BMI = \frac{Weight\ in\ Pounds}{(Height\ in\ inches) \times (Height\ in\ inches)} \times 703$$

A woman's BMI is always based on her prepregnancy weight and is the gold standard in weight evaluation (although BMI calculations do not take into account factors such as build, which can influence a person's weight). Knowing how much someone weighs doesn't mean a lot unless you know how tall she is and can compare the two numbers.

A BMI of 20 to 25 is considered "normal." A BMI of 27 to 30 is considered "overweight," and a BMI of more than 30 is considered "obese." A BMI of more than 35 or 40 is sometimes called "morbidly obese." To get an idea of what these numbers mean, consider a woman who is five feet, five inches tall. If she weighed 175 pounds, she would be considered overweight. If she weighed 190 pounds, she would be considered obese. If she weighed 240 pounds, she would be considered morbidly obese.

Doctors and scientists use these terms in their studies, and we'll use them in this chapter in the same way, even though the terms may seem offensive. Remember, they are just words. Use them to understand the information provided, then push them out of your mind. You don't need to hang a label on yourself.

The results of medical studies can sometimes be confusing because of the groups they consider. One study might only calculate the risk for "overweight" women for a certain condition, while another might only calculate the risk for "obese" women. If a study finds a risk for overweight women, you can infer that obese women have a similar risk (since obese women weigh more than overweight women, they would have at least the same amount of risk). But if a study finds a risk for obese women, you can't assume that it means overweight women are also at risk (because overweight women weigh less, and it's possible that their weight is not at a level where it has an impact on the condition being described).

"I had the opportunity to read a report from my second-level ultrasound, and I was embarrassed and insulted to see myself described as "moderately obese." It was my first pregnancy and I weighed more before I got pregnant than I wanted to, but still, to see myself described that way really hurt my feelings and made me feel awful about myself. I did a little research and found out it was a medical term. That made me feel better—a little."—Lee T.

Polycystic Ovarian Syndrome (PCOS)

PCOS (also sometimes called Syndrome O) is a medical condition in which a woman is often obese, hirsute (or hairy), has polycystic ovaries

(ovaries which develop small fluid-filled cysts), has irregular menstrual cycles, may not ovulate, and experiences infertility problems. PCOS patients also often have insulin resistance, which contributes to their infertility. Many women with PCOS are undiagnosed, and it is estimated that 5 to 10 percent of women have this condition. If you think that this description fits you, you should discuss it with your health-care provider.

PCOS is of concern in pregnancy because it can lead to miscarriage. PCOS patients with infertility may be given a diabetes drug called Metformin (Glucophage) as part of their treatment even though they don't have diabetes. This drug helps to increase fertility and reduce the miscarriage rate. The drug is usually stopped once ultrasound confirms a pregnancy, but in some circumstances, the woman may stay on it for the entire pregnancy. Glucophage is safe during the first trimester of pregnancy and doesn't cause birth defects. Women with PCOS are at a high risk for the development of diabetes and gestational diabetes.

You can have a successful pregnancy with PCOS—the hard part for many women is getting pregnant. Talk about your condition with your health-care provider, and arm yourself with information.

If you are concerned about PCOS, the Polycystic Ovarian Syndrome Association has information on its Web site at *www.pscosa.org*. They also have an online quiz you can take to gauge how likely it is that you might have this disorder at *www.pcosupport.org/support/quiz.php*.

"I had a series of recurrent miscarriage tests done after my second miscarriage. After I learned about my PCOS, I was convinced I would never carry another baby to term. I was told that women with PCOS were in a higher-risk category for miscarriage. My doctor treated my last pregnancy as high risk. Testing showed I had antiphospholipid syndrome (blood clotting disorder) so I was put on a baby aspirin a day. I also tested in the low range of normal for my progesterone, so I took 200 mg of prometrium a day until fourteen weeks. At thirty weeks, I went for weekly nonstress tests to make sure everything was OK with the baby."—Amy S.

Pregnancy Conditions

Gestational Diabetes

Gestational diabetes is a condition in which the pregnant mother's body doesn't produce enough insulin (a chemical that allows our bodies to digest sugar or glucose) or is unable to use the insulin it has (known as insulin resistance). When the body doesn't have enough insulin or isn't using its insulin properly, sugar (glucose) accumulates throughout the body and can cause damage to internal organs, eyes, nerves, and blood vessels. A 2003 study by the National Institute of Child Health and Human Development (NICHD) showed that the incidence of gestational diabetes in normal-weight women was 2.3 percent, in obese women 6.3 percent, and in morbidly obese women 9.5 percent.

Normal pregnancy requires the mother to make more insulin and for the insulin to work effectively. Some women are unable to meet this need. The reason for this may be genetic, related to weight, age, or a combination of these factors (so if you get it, you can't assume it's just because you're overweight). These women develop an increase in their blood-glucose level, usually after meals and, at times, when fasting. This is usually seen in the second half of pregnancy (after twenty to twenty-four weeks).

Gestational diabetes does not usually cause blood-sugar elevation comparable to regular (overt) diabetes. In fact, the blood-glucose levels of women with gestational diabetes wouldn't qualify them to be categorized as diabetics were they not pregnant. However, if not controlled, elevated blood-sugar levels can cause problems for the baby.

Pre-pregnancy (overt) diabetes can be associated with an increased risk of birth defects such as neural tube defects and congenital heart disease. The risk has to do with poor sugar control and high sugar levels during the first trimester. If you are diabetic it is important to discuss this with your health-care provider. Most cases of gestational diabetes develop later in pregnancy and carry a much lower risk of birth defects. Gestational diabetes occurs predominantly in the second half of pregnancy (after twenty to twenty-four weeks). This type of gestational diabetes is the most common and is not associated with an increased risk of birth defects or congenital anomalies. Some women have evidence of gestational diabetes in early pregnancy or have blood-sugar elevations that would be equivalent to a nonpregnant woman with regular (overt) diabetes. In these women, it's likely that they had undetected impaired-glucose intolerance or diabetes before they became pregnant, which was discovered only during the pregnancy. In these pregnancies, there is an increased risk of birth defects.

The message here is to get tested for diabetes before pregnancy if you or your health-care provider believe you are at risk because preconception care will control these risks. Of course, chances are, if you're reading this book, you are already pregnant, and this news is coming a bit late. It is recommended that you be tested yearly for diabetes if your health-care provider believes you are at risk and if you have a family history.

If you find out that you have diabetes early in your pregnancy, don't panic, work with your health-care provider to get it under control and undergo necessary testing. It's very likely that your health-care provider will be able to help you control your condition and you will have a healthy baby.

The biggest risk with gestational diabetes is having an oversized or large baby, usually defined as over nine pounds (called a large-for-gestational-age baby). A large baby can mean difficulties with delivery, but because C-sections are an option, this is not even close to being the end of the world. (Read more details about large babies in Chapter 16.) If diabetes is not well controlled during pregnancy, the newborn can experience breathing problems, jaundice (a treatable liver problem that causes a slight yellowing of the skin), and low blood sugar (again, this is treatable). In a small percent of cases, gestational diabetes is also associated with an increased risk for stillbirth (but these cases are usually ones requiring insulin treatment where sugar control is poor, so if you are getting good medical care, you shouldn't worry), preterm labor, and problems with amniotic-fluid levels. Another problem is neonatal hypocalcemia (low calcium level in newborns), which is treatable and self-limiting. You should understand, though, that these problems are not common, and the biggest worry doctors have about gestational diabetes is the size of the baby, which just means you may end up having a C-section. There is also some evidence that babies whose mothers had gestational diabetes are more likely to be overweight as adults.

It's important to understand that all of these problems usually occur when the mother's diabetes is not well controlled. If it is controlled, the baby's risk is very small.

Gestational diabetes is diagnosed with a blood test (after drinking a glucose drink and waiting one hour), normally between week twenty-four and week twenty-eight of pregnancy. If your results are high, you'll probably be sent for a three-hour test, which is considered the gold standard for diagnosis. Some health-care providers test overweight women earlier in pregnancy because they are at a higher risk for undiagnosed diabetes prior to pregnancy. Because there is a higher risk to the baby with early pregnancy diabetes, this can be a good idea if you haven't been tested recently.

Standard glucose testing occurs in the second trimester. If you pass it but have borderline results, your health-care provider may wish to have you tested again in the third trimester. Note that there is usually no reason to be tested monthly or biweekly. If your health-care provider recommends this, ask the reasons. If he is concerned that you are high risk or borderline, it might make more sense to follow a gestational diabetes diet instead of putting yourself through the constant testing. Discuss these options with your provider.

Mothers with gestational diabetes need to control their blood-sugar level with diet and exercise. Blood sugar testing is performed first thing in the morning (called a fasting glucose test) and usually one or two hours after each meal. Some doctors will only test blood sugar periodically. Most women with gestational diabetes test their own blood sugar at home using a glucometer on a daily basis. Diet and exercise will control blood sugar, but a small percentage of women may need additional treatment with insulin or an oral medication called Glyburide. Some women with PCOS may use Metformin.(To learn more about a gestational diabetes diet and about diabetes in general, contact the American Diabetes Association at *www.diabetes.org/gestational-diabetes.jsp* or by calling 800-342-2383.) The baby's size will be carefully monitored, and nonstress tests may be advised later in pregnancy to monitor the baby's heart rate.

According to the American Diabetes Association, two out of three women with gestational diabetes will have the condition again in later pregnancies. If you have gestational diabetes, there is also an increased risk (50 percent) for developing type 2 diabetes within five to ten years after your pregnancy. Because of this, it's important to get tested yearly after a gestational diabetes pregnancy. Remember, gestational diabetes can be controlled through diet and exercise and when well controlled, the risk to mother and baby is small. If you are diagnosed with gestational diabetes, you might want to ask for a referral to a nutritionist or dietician.

"I was borderline for gestational diabetes so I didn't actually have GD, but I had to watch what I ate. And I visited a registered dietician to see how I could maximize my nutrition while being lactose intolerant and having food allergies. I was careful about what I ate in the sense that I avoided lots of candy or processed sugar, and I only ate fruit with meals."—DeAnn R.

"I have PCOS and am insulin resistant. I was taking Glucophage when I got pregnant and decided I wanted to stay on through much of my pregnancy. In order to do this, the doctors said I must follow their guidelines. They told me that being that overweight and already insulin resistant, there was no way I wouldn't develop gestational diabetes. So, the first thing I had to do was meet the diabetes specialists, and they showed me how to test my blood sugar (four times a day). Then I had to meet with the nutritionist where I was given the diet. I also had my first gestational diabetes test at twenty weeks, then again at twenty-four and twenty-eight. They constantly came back normal. Also at this time, I was having an ultrasound and nonstress test every week because that was their protocol for GD patients. At thirty-two weeks, they decided I needed to go for the three-hour test even though I passed all the one-hour tests. This, too, came back normal. However, they continued to make me do the ultrasounds and NSTs. I was a nervous wreck! They made me feel like I was doomed, and I was destined to have a horrible pregnancy, and my child would suffer because of my health. I blame all my terrible feelings and memories on them forcing me into following the GD protocol."—Heather G.

Preeclampsia

If you experience high blood pressure after the twentieth week of pregnancy and have no prior history of hypertension, you are described as having gestational hypertension (some physicians use the term pregnancy-induced hypertension or "PIH," but this is considered outdated).

Hypertension may be a warning sign of the disorder called preeclampsia. Preeclampsia is a condition that includes high blood pressure, protein in the urine, and edema (swelling). Between 5 and 10 percent of all pregnant women experience preeclampsia. Obese women have their risk increased by 3.5 times. Women who have high blood pressure prior to pregnancy are at higher risk for developing this condition, as well. It is most common in first pregnancies and usually occurs after the twentieth week.

Some studies show that taking vitamin E and C during pregnancy may help prevent preeclampsia, especially in women at risk. The doses were high—1,000 mg vitamin C and 400 IU vitamin E daily. Low-dose aspirin (81 mg) daily during pregnancy may also help prevent preeclampsia, but ONLY in women at high risk for the disorder. Obesity by itself is not considered a reason for these treatments. It may make sense for a larger woman to take low-dose aspirin during pregnancy if she has hypertension before she becomes pregnant, but you should NOT self-medicate. Find out what your health-care provider recommends.

Severe preeclampsia can lead to central nervous system problems (blurred vision, headaches, confusion), stroke, and kidney failure. A serious condition called HELLP syndrome can occur which can lead to liver failure, severe anemia (low blood count), and blood clotting deficiency. Preeclampsia can lead to eclampsia, a serious condition involving seizures, which can be life-threatening for the pregnant woman. Severe preeclampsia and eclampsia are relatively rare conditions. Preeclampsia and eclampsia usually end at delivery. Induction of labor can be a solution in severe cases, but only if the baby is developed enough. Some drugs are considered safe for treatment during pregnancy.

Most pregnant women experience some edema during pregnancy, and this does *not* mean you are developing preeclampsia. Drinking a lot of water and wearing support hose can help, but you should talk to your health-care provider about your particular situation. If you are diagnosed with hypertension or preeclampsia, talk with your provider about the steps you can take to stay healthy. In severe cases, bed rest may be necessary.

"They assumed I would have gestational diabetes and preeclampsia since I was so big. My sugars were perfect, and my BP was perfect until a week before I gave birth."—Julie M.

"I had pregnancy-induced high blood pressure with my first and am trying really hard not to get it with my second. I was put on complete bed rest for the last month of my pregnancy. At first, I did not realize that being overweight attributed to my high BP."—Shannan E.

"I had high blood pressure with all three pregnancies, and it was very scary. I was concerned for myself, as well as my babies. I was put on moderate bed rest toward the end of all three pregnancies and had labor induced each time because of my high blood pressure. Somewhere in the back of my mind I wondered if I had taken better care of myself would I still have had this problem with my blood pressure, but I know of other women who are normal weight and still had problems. In the end, everything worked out, and that's all that matters."—Beth U.

"My blood pressure became an issue toward the end of my pregnancy. I spent the last two weeks on bed rest."—Vanessa R.

"Preeclampsia in both pregnancies. My feet swelled up like balloons, forcing me to bed rest and to keep my feet elevated as much as possible. This was hard as I'm an active person, but I realized how serious the situation was for me and my baby."—Sharon L.

Preterm Birth

Preterm birth (or birth before full gestational age) occurs before the thirty-seventh week of pregnancy. Preterm birth occurs in 11.6 percent of all births. There is no link between being overweight and going into preterm labor. However, if you have gestational diabetes, preeclampsia, or hypertension, your risk is elevated.

Urinary Tract Infections (UTIs)

There is evidence that obese women have a higher incidence of urinary tract infections during pregnancy. And because of the changes to the kidneys during pregnancy, there is a tendency for UTIs to spread to the kidneys, causing kidney infections. Untreated UTIs can lead to preterm labor. If you feel like you have to go to the bathroom all the time (and yes, this is a very common symptom of pregnancy, so it can be impossible to know it's caused by a UTI), feel like you aren't going to make it to the bathroom in time, or have pain or burning during urination, let your health-care provider know. Urinary tract infections are easily treated. Many women get urinary tract infections without realizing it because they don't experience any of the common symptoms. (This is called an asymptomatic infection.) It is recommended that plus-size pregnant women have their urine tested once every three months for an asymptomatic infection.

"I had a bladder infection with symptoms that included painful urination (burning), low-grade fever, and some right-sided kidney pain. The treatment was 500 mg, two times a day, of amoxicillin. I was worried about taking medication of any kind while pregnant, but the OB assured me that amox was safe for the baby. After that, I drank more water, drank cranberry juice, and urinated after intercourse. I didn't get another one."—Beth U.

Sleep Apnea

Sleep apnea happens when the tissue surrounding a windpipe (larynx) causes it to open and close during sleep, leading to drop in the body's oxygen level. It is common in people who are overweight or obese. It may cause loud snoring, sudden awakening, feeling tired or fatigued in the daytime, and depression. There is some evidence that sleep apnea during pregnancy may have effects on the baby, causing low birth weight or even stillbirth. Notify your health-care provider if you have any of these symptoms. It can be diagnosed with sleep studies and treated with continuous-positive-airway-pressure (CPAP) oxygen therapy at home. If you have already been diagnosed with obstructive sleep apnea, you should see a perinatal specialist before and during pregnancy.

Miscarriage

Being overweight does not increase your risk for miscarriage. It is difficult to pinpoint exactly what the overall rate of miscarriage is since many miscarriages happen within the first one or two weeks of pregnancy before the pregnancy is known. Some sources say that up to 50 percent of all conceptions end in miscarriage. During weeks three to six of pregnancy, the general miscarriage rate is 10 percent. From six to 12 weeks, it is 5 percent. Once the baby's heartbeat has been detected, miscarriage rate drops to 2 percent among all pregnancies. Several studies have examined the miscarriage rate for obese women following fertility treatments, and the rate has been reported at 27 percent. This applies only to fertility treatment cases and may not take into account the fact mentioned above that 50 percent of all early pregnancies end in what are usually unknown miscarriages. During fertility treatments, pregnancy is usually detected very early so it can be monitored closely, thus more of these early miscarriages are probably detected.

"I had a miscarriage with my third pregnancy. The thing with early miscarriage is that you can never know what caused it. The doctor told me that it most likely was because there was something genetically wrong with the baby and that probably more than 50 percent of all pregnancies end in miscarriage. I can't help wondering if somehow my weight was responsible."—Lee T.

"My mother has always hinted to the fact that my weight had something to do with my losses, but testing would prove her wrong."—Amy S.

Birth Complications

Overweight and obese women are thirteen times more likely than average women to experience overdue birth, longer labor, induced labor, and blood loss during labor, according to the American Obesity Association. Most of these conditions can be managed and cared for by your health-care provider, so none of them are the end of the world.

Due to the increased incidence of larger babies in larger women, delivery can be complicated. The most common complication with a large baby is shoulder dystocia. This occurs when the baby's head emerges from the birth canal, but the shoulders, usually because they are so large, are stuck. There is the risk of a broken arm or clavicle for the baby, as well as nerve damage. Larger babies can also mean larger episiotomies, vaginal lacerations, and blood loss for mothers during delivery.

While this sounds frightening, most providers know in advance if you are going to have a very large baby and can take steps to ensure labor will be successful or can recommend a C-section if necessary. It's also important to remember that women of all sizes deliver large babies every day, and size does not mean you will have birth complications. Most large babies are delivered successfully, although you can be sure that people will relish telling you horror stories!

Stillbirth

Stillbirth (medically defined as the death of the fetus after the twentieth week of pregnancy) occurs in half of one percent of all births according to the March of Dimes. Overweight and obese women are known to have an increased risk roughly double this, equal to about 1 percent, and these tend to happen in the third trimester. The risk seems to be highest for women who have morbid obesity, and medical science does not quite understand why. If you are very overweight, your health-care provider may want to do weekly or twice weekly fetal monitoring and additional ultrasounds in the third trimester to keep an eye on things. The risk of stillbirth is very small, and if you are receiving good pregnancy care, it's not something you should worry about.

Twins

Obese women are 2.1 times more likely to have fraternal twins than smaller women. Additionally, women who are taller than five feet, five inches are 1.7 times more likely. So if you're tall, your chance may be increased. If you're carrying twins, you'll need to gain more weight, and your health-care provider may recommend that you gain twenty to twenty-five pounds, but be sure to ask what is recommended in your situation.

It's not clear why plus-size women are more likely to have twins, but it probably has something to do with a higher level of LH and FSH hormones (the hormones that stimulate ovulation), which causes the ovaries to produce more than one egg at a time. Additionally, since some plus-size women have difficulty conceiving (particularly if they have PCOS), they may be placed on fertility drugs such as Clomiphene, which can lead to the development of multiple eggs.

Having twins may increase your risk for hypertension or gestational diabetes, and twins may come earlier or result in a more-complicated delivery, so be sure to talk with your health-care provider if you discover you have two wonderful babies growing inside you instead of just one.

Effect on the Baby
Birth Defects

A birth defect is defined by the March of Dimes as "an abnormality of structure, function or metabolism (body chemistry) present at birth that results in physical or mental disability, or is fatal." This definition sounds frightening, but what it's saying is that a birth defect is abnormal development that causes the child to face some kind of disability (which can range from mild to severe). There are more than 4,000 types of birth defects that have been categorized. Genes cause many, many birth defects. Others are related to environment (such as exposure to drugs or chemicals). The weight of the mother is considered to be an environmental factor. Still other birth defects result from a combination of gene abnormalities and environment. Medical science does not completely understand birth defects or all of their origins. It's important to realize that birth defects usually can't be pinned on something specific like the mother's weight, although there are studies that can show increased risk for overweight women for certain defects.

A 2003 report from the Centers for Disease Control (CDC) showed that women who were overweight were twice as likely as average women to have a baby with a major defect. However, the results of this study aren't quite as alarming when you consider that average-weight women are at a 3- to 5-percent risk for having a baby with a major birth defect, and overweight and obese women are at a 6- to 10-percent risk. A contrasting study from the March of Dimes shows that babies of both overweight and obese women are at only a 1.4-percent risk of a major birth defect. Clearly more research needs to be done, but you should talk to your doctor or midwife about the risks.

There are several types of birth defects that have separately defined risk factors.

Omphalocele

This is a birth defect in which the baby's abdominal organs protrude through his or her navel. Average women are at a 1-percent risk (a contrasting study reported this as only a 1 in 5000 risk), and a recent CDC study showed obese women to have 3.3 times the risk of average weight women. Omphalocele is associated with elevated maternal-serum-alpha-fetoprotein levels (diagnosed by the triple or multiscreen test early in pregnancy). Getting this test can help flag this condition. Underweight women are also at risk for this disorder, so it may have links to poor nutrition. Eating healthy may be a way to reduce the risk. Discuss this with your doctor or midwife.

Heart Defects

One in every 125 to 150 babies is born with heart defects. For overweight and obese women, the risk is doubled, according to a CDC study, to two in every 125 to 150 babies. Parents who have a child with heart abnormalities are at an increased risk to have later children with heart defects. And parents who have a heart defect are at a higher risk of having a child with a problem. If you fit either of these two scenarios, talk to your doctor or midwife about your elevated risk. You may be referred to a genetic counselor. Some defects can be detected with ultra-sounds. If a problem is suspected in the ultrasound, the mother may be referred for a specialized ultrasound called an echocardiograph, which can more accurately detect heart problems.

Avoiding alcohol and drugs during pregnancy can help ensure your baby will be born with a normal heart. Talk to your doctor or midwife for more details. Many heart defects can be surgically repaired in the first two years of life.

"My daughter was born with pulmonary stenosis, and though no one said it was related to my weight, I wondered. This is a heart defect that causes an obstruction in the blood flowing to and/or from the heart. No one in my family had this defect, and I couldn't help but feel responsible. Was it caused by something I did wrong during a critical stage of pregnancy? Since she was diagnosed with this at birth, I had access to the hospital pediatric cardiologist who took the time to answer all of my questions. For me, understanding the defect and how it would affect my daughter's life was the best way to cope. Unfortunately from what I learned, I felt even more responsible. Statistically, children born to overweight moms have a much-higher incidence of heart defects. Fortunately, she had a mild case of pulmonary stenosis, and as she grew, her condition improved. By her third year, the defect had repaired itself, and she was given a clean bill of health. If your child has a birth defect, I think it is important to learn everything you can about how this affects your child's quality of life, how it will change your family dynamics, and what you CAN do to make a difference."—Beth T.

Open Neural-tube Defects

Neural-tube defects are abnormalities that have to do with the neural tube, an early formation in the baby that develops into the spine and brain. There are lots of conflicting reports when it comes to neural-tube defects and its relation to the mother's weight. Studies in the journals *Fetal Diagnostic Therapy* and *Epidemiology* both concluded that there is *no* increased risk to overweight or obese women. Other studies have placed overweight women at an increased risk of 1.9 times or 3 times that of average weight women.

There are many types of open neural tube defects. The two most common are anencephaly and spina bifida. Spina bifida causes a portion of the spinal cord to be exposed on the baby's back. Usually the spinal cord below the exposed portion does not function properly and many of these babies also have brain problems such as hydrocephalus (sometimes called water on the brain). Depending on the severity, paralysis can occur, but some children with mild cases have no symptoms or mild symptoms. The average woman has a risk of one in 2,000. A recent CDC study indicates that obese women are at 3.5 times the risk for babies with spina bifida (so, remember, this means only 3.5 out of 2000). Parents who have one child with the disorder are at a much-higher risk that later children will also have it. This disorder can be detected with the maternal serum alphafetoprotein test (triple-screen test). Spina bifida is treatable with surgery. High temperature baths or steam rooms such as are found in saunas or health club whirlpool baths should be avoided during pregnancy since high temperatures can cause birth defects such as spina bifida in the first trimester. For more information about spina bifida, contact the Spina Bifida Association of America at *www.sbaa.org* or 800-621-3141.

Anencephaly is another type of open neural-tube defect in which the baby is born without essential parts of the brain. This occurs in one in 1,000 births. The risk for overweight women is doubled, to two in 1,000.

Neural-tube defects have gotten a lot of press in the last ten years because studies have shown that taking folic-acid supplements three months before and during the first twelve weeks of pregnancy can drastically reduce the occurrence of neural-tube defects. However, a study in the *Journal of the American Medical Association* has shown that folic acid does not have the same preventive effect in overweight women (at least not at the dosages recommended for average-weight women). There is speculation that perhaps overweight women need to take a larger dose of folic acid to get the preventive benefits. The usual dose of preconception folate recommended for all women is 400 micrograms or 0.4 mg daily for at least three months prior to conception and continuing until twelve-weeks gestation. Since folate is a harmless vitamin it might make sense to be given the higher dose, 4 mg per day, using the same time period as is used for the usual dose. This may be given by prescription or some health-food stores may have folate in strengths of 1 to 2 mg, and several pills could be taken to reach the 4-mg mark. You should discuss your folate intake with your health-care provider and make a decision with his or her recommendation. There is also some evidence that multivitamins are beneficial. However, avoid megadoses of vitamins, especially the fat-soluble vitamins A and D, since megadoses of these vitamins may cause birth defects. Avoidance of alcohol, tobacco, and any type of illicit substances is essential.

Screening for open neural-tube defects is generally done between fifteen and eighteen weeks using a blood test called the maternal serum alpha-fetoprotein (MSAFP). Sometimes two or three additional hormones are added to the test to screen for fetal chromosome problems, and the test is then called the "triple screen" or the "quadruple screen." Your weight will be recorded on the laboratory requisition since adjustments for weight must be made by the lab for the test to be accurate. Don't be surprised or offended when you are weighed or asked your weight when you go to have blood drawn. The alpha-fetoprotein is what is used to detect open neural-tube defects and is elevated in their presence. The test detects 85 percent of spina bifidas and 90 to 95 percent of anencephaly. There are many reasons for an elevated level, and an elevated level does not necessarily mean there is an open neural-tube defect or anything wrong. If your test results show an elevated level, don't panic and jump to conclusions. This test should be thought of as a screening test that identifies patients who need to proceed to the next level of testing, either a high-resolution ultrasound or amniocentesis.

Ultrasound is somewhat more sensitive and detects 90 to 95 percent of spina bifida and 100 percent of anencephaly. One or both tests may be ordered depending on your personal risk.

Multiple Birth Defects

The term multiple birth defects simply means that a baby is born with one or more abnormalities. Of babies born with birth defects, between 20 and 30 percent have multiple defects. The risk for overweight women is double that of average women.

Birth Weight

Large babies are often associated with larger women, particularly those who experience gestational diabetes. Between 16 and 30 percent of babies born to obese women are macrosomic, or large (weighing more than nine pounds), compared to 10 percent of total pregnancies. Large babies are usually healthy, but problems may arise during delivery, as discussed earlier.

But here is some good news about plus-size pregnancies! The larger a woman's prepregnancy weight, the smaller the chance that her baby will have low birth weight.

"The baby was big. I felt guilty about getting pregnant when I already had this weight problem. But, of course, the baby doesn't care."—Liz R.

Coping with Your Risk

Now that you've read—and maybe been made to feel nervous—about your risk, first put it in perspective. None of these statistics indicate that any of these things will happen to you or your baby. You have excellent odds (not many people would want to bet that you would face these conditions based on the odds) and will most likely have a beautiful, healthy baby and an uneventful pregnancy.

If you feel a little nervous at the prospect of the things described in this chapter, the best thing you can do is be proactive. Talk to your doctor or midwife about your pregnancy, ask questions about your increased risk, make sure you are tested for gestational diabetes and that you get an ultrasound during pregnancy. Find out about other tests (such as the triple screen or quad screen), and follow your care provider's advice about exercise and nutrition.

While knowledge is a good thing, excessive worrying is not. Worrying is not going to help you avoid pregnancy complications—it's just going to make you feel worse about everything. Resolve right now to gather information, and be honest with your care provider, but don't let this dominate your life or your pregnancy. Get the facts, ask questions, process the information, and then push it aside. If your care provider gives you advice about steps you can take to help reduce your risk, follow them, but don't obsess about the chances of this or that happening.

Pregnancy is a very emotional time for most women. Things that might seem small at other times can seem overwhelming during pregnancy. It's perfectly OK to express your feelings, your fears, and your worries to your partner, your caregiver, close family, and friends. You don't have to repress what you're experiencing. What you do need to do is find a way to work through it and let go of it. You might worry throughout your entire pregnancy about your baby's health (and remember that *all* women do this), but you can't let it consume you.

Weight-Control Drugs and Procedures

In recent years, more and more options have become available to people who want medical assistance losing weight. While these truly do work miracles for some people, it's important to understand how they impact pregnancy.

There are two prescription weight-loss drugs currently in use. Sibutramine is an appetite suppressant. Orlistat is a drug that decreases the body's ability to absorb fat. Both are known to help people lose weight. If you are taking these drugs and wish to become pregnant, it is a good idea to go off them several months before trying to conceive. You should never take these drugs while pregnant because the risk to an unborn baby has not been studied. If you are taking or have taken these drugs, consult your health-care provider for more information.

Over-the-counter appetite suppressant drugs, supplements, and foods are also not considered safe for use during pregnancy. If you are taking and would like to become pregnant, it is a good idea to stop using them several months before trying to conceive.

Another popular weight-control measure is bariatric surgery. There are two types of bariatric surgeries. In gastric bypass, the lower end of the stomach is detached from its usual connection to the small bowel and implanted lower down the gastrointestinal tract. This bypasses, or goes around, parts of the small bowel that are involved in the digestion and absorption of food, resulting in fewer calories absorbed and weight loss. The problem with this type of surgery is that vital nutrients such as iron, and B vitamins (especially B-12) are not absorbed, and fat absorption may be limited. For this reason, gastric bypass is also called "malabsorptive surgery." Outcomes for pregnancies in which the mother had this surgery before she became pregnant are generally good. Mothers sometimes develop severe iron deficiency and may need iron to be given intramuscularly or intravenously. Vitamin B-12 shots must also be administered. During the postpartum period, some of these patients have decreased fat content in their breast milk, which may also be a problem. However, the general outcome for the baby is good, and with proper care, most women in this category do well. There is evidence that pregnancy risks are highest in the first year after the surgery, particularly concerning poor fetal growth. Generally, it is best to avoid pregnancy for the first year after this procedure.

The other type of bariatric surgery is gastric banding. This surgery involves making the stomach smaller by "banding," while keeping it connected to the small bowel naturally. This restricts calories without having problems with malabsorption. For this reason, this type of surgery is called a "restrictive procedure." A newer form of this is the adjustable gastric banding, which is done through a laparoscope (a small operating instrument that does not require a large surgical incision). A band is placed around the stomach, and it can be adjusted using tubing or a port, which is on the skin. Adjustments of the band can be made according to the patient's weight-loss needs. There have been several pregnancies with this type of band, and so far they have been largely successful.

There is evidence that women who undergo bariatric surgery lower their risks for hypertension, gestational diabetes, C-section, and large babies. And the resulting weight loss can greatly increase fertility. If you have had bariatric surgery, it is essential that you discuss it with your health-care provider. If you are considering bariatric surgery after your pregnancy, you should wait until you finish breastfeeding or until your health care provider gives you the go-ahead.

8

Feeling Good About Your Body

The best way to maintain a positive attitude throughout your pregnancy is to feel good about your body and yourself as a person. This may sound like a tall order, but it really is possible to love, appreciate, and care for your body—even if you can't stand the thought of gaining another pound, hate looking in the mirror, or believe the talk about beauty during pregnancy is nonsense. Finding ways to see beauty in yourself will give you more confidence and help you feel comfortable in your own skin.

"Pamper, pamper, pamper! Whatever makes you feel better."—Vanessa R.

"One thing about babies, they don't care how their mom looks. Mom is all good things. So be mom, enjoy the baby, and your own role as nurturer. I haven't experienced anything in life nearly as satisfying as being pregnant and having babies. That's why I've done it so many times."—Liz R.

Changing Your Attitude

First you must tackle your beliefs and attitudes about your body. Most of these have been pressed upon you by society and the prejudices of others. Recognize that these negative feelings stem from outside sources. You need to be able to free yourself from these feelings.

Think about your body like a unique piece of art. You simply can't compare a Picasso to a Monet, so there's no reason to believe you should compare your body to your size-8 sister-in-law or your size-10 friend who is also pregnant. Beauty and value in life are not about size. A sunflower and a lily of the valley are vastly different in size, but one is not better than the other. Both have beauty and value, and both have special and wonderful qualities.

Your body was beautiful before you became pregnant (just ask your partner!), and it is even more beautiful now that it is pregnant. Look at your body objectively, without being weighed down by societal constraints. Appreciate its curves, softness, colors, proportion, and movements. There is so much to love and value if you open your eyes.

You must stop evaluating yourself as "fat" or "huge" or in any other way with regard to size. Stop comparing yourself to others and start seeing that what you have is beautiful.

"When it's just my naked body and the mirror, I feel beautiful. I can appreciate what my husband likes about my body. But once I put on clothes, forget it. Once in a while if I have a terrific outfit, then I can feel good, but most of the time, I just don't."—Karen K.

"Love yourself, no matter what. If you are unhappy with yourself, you may start to 'blame' the baby, and that's not fair. Giving life is a miracle! And a few pounds and stretch marks are really a small price to pay for the joys motherhood brings. It's just fat, it will go away! Be healthy, eat right, but don't make yourself miserable. Remember, if mama ain't happy, ain't nobody happy."—Vanessa R.

Appreciating Your Miracle

Pregnancy is a miracle. You already know this and have felt it from the beginning. You may tend to dismiss it, since your growing baby is now a fact of your everyday life, but take a minute, and really consider what is happening. Your body has taken microscopic pieces and caused them to grow into what will be a complete and perfect human being. Inside your tummy, you are carrying, nurturing, and creating a child that will forever be linked to you. It is truly magical and miraculous that your body can perform this feat.

Your pregnant body is the outward demonstration of what is happening inside you. An entire human being is developing inside your abdomen. Of course your stomach is going to start to look bigger! Of course your body is going to change shape and make adjustments. Your body must adapt to accommodate this new life.

It can be disconcerting to watch these changes happen completely outside of your control. To have a stomach, hips, and breasts you have been taught to believe are too large to begin with, increase in size can feel quite depressing. If you felt fat before, you probably feel positively humongous now. You may feel disgusted with the changes, worried about being able to reverse them, and completely devoid of attractiveness.

First, you must remember that these changes happen to all women during pregnancy, regardless of size. It is simply the nature of pregnancy. The changes are necessary and part of a stunning biological transformation. Your body is doing exactly what it's supposed to, and needs to, do. Stop trying to fight it. Your body is pretty darn smart to know how to do all these complicated maneuvers so that your baby can grow and be born.

Your pregnancy is a brief period, a short moment in your life, really. Going through it embarrassed, depressed, and self-conscious is no way to celebrate and enjoy this incredible miracle. Consider everything your body is doing, and feel proud! Your growing tummy and widening hips are part of an amazing process. The changes you are going through only serve to make your already wonderful body stunningly beautiful.

Don't be ashamed of the wonderful curves and lovely roundness pregnancy brings. Rejoice in them, revel in them, and proudly stand up and carry them each day.

"I just accepted what was going on and decided to look forward to my plan of losing weight later. I just wanted to do the best I could for my baby, to have a healthy pregnancy in the hope that it would mean an easier birth and healthy baby. That was the main thing for me."—Amanda F.

Pampering Yourself

Taking the time to pamper and care for your body will help you enjoy it, appreciate it, and give it the respect and awe it deserves. And if you can appreciate and respect your body, you will find that you feel good about yourself and how you look. Make time to do things that feel good to your body and make you feel good about your body. This can be as simple as taking the time for a bath instead of a shower, putting up your feet when you are sitting, or splurging a little.

Make a point of treating yourself to something that feels wonderful or makes you feel good about yourself at least once a week. Try some of these suggestions for ways to pamper your beautiful pregnant body:

Personal Care
- purchase different scented lotions
- take long bubble baths
- try bath beads or bath oil
- experiment with new makeup: colors, brands, types, etc. or have a professional do your face
- get a new haircut
- color or perm your hair (once your health-care provider feels it's safe)
- try new hairstyles at home
- exfoliate

- sample new perfumes and splurge on one that makes you feel great
- get a professional manicure or pedicure
- try a new shower gel
- buy lotion for specific body parts, e.g. feet, elbows, cuticles, forehead, and so on
- gently massage your tummy with baby oil
- have your legs waxed
- pluck your eyebrows
- clean your pores with a nose strip
- give your hair a hot-oil treatment
- try some nail decals or an exciting new nail polish color
- buy a foot spa

Your Surroundings

- purchase a bath pillow
- use sheets with high thread count for a luxurious feeling
- try satin sheets
- add extra pillows to your bed
- get a down comforter or a lightweight quilt
- buy or find a pillow or footstool to rest your feet on when you are sitting
- use huge fluffy bath towels in your favorite color
- light scented candles or use potpourri to enhance your environment
- buy or rent a portable whirlpool maker for your tub
- claim the most comfortable chair in the living room or family room as your own
- order healthy take-out once in a while instead of cooking
- rent movies and curl up to watch them
- treat yourself to an expensive restaurant meal
- buy something that will make your life easier, like a laptop or a new dishwasher

Clothing and Accessories

- wear jewelry you love
- buy one gorgeous, expensive outfit for yourself, and wear it
- buy clothing that feels pleasing to your skin and is not tight or constraining
- wear silky lingerie
- buy new costume jewelry to dress up your maternity outfits
- cuddle up in flannel and fluffy slippers on cold nights
- dress up your outfits with scarves and accessories
- get a new pair of sunglasses
- choose pretty underwear
- wear big, soft, comfortable socks

All of these ideas will help you focus on yourself while making you feel absolutely wonderful. Make the time to do little things for yourself, and you will find that you appreciate your body more and feel better about it.

"I didn't feel good about myself and I didn't do enough for myself. That was a mistake."—Heather E.

"I got regular pedicures. This helped with my edema, as well as achy feet. It also helped me feel pretty and feminine while I was in a body that didn't always feel like it still belonged to me. I took long, leisurely baths and did my hair and makeup regularly, mostly because I knew once I gave birth, I wouldn't have time for me. So I pampered myself while I had the time."—Vanessa R.

"Most massage-therapy clinics have the pregnancy pillow, allowing even expectant moms to enjoy a much-needed rubdown."—Dana C.

"I did keep my toenails painted, as well as my nails."—Tammy M.

"Friday nights were reserved for a nice bath and facial mask. I used to also give myself a pedicure, but that became impossible after a time as I couldn't see my feet, let alone reach them."—Sharon L.

"I just loved lying about in the bath and watching TV. Most of the time, I felt pretty revolting because of my weight and morning sickness. Those lovely baths in the early evening really helped me feel more human. I also loved getting my nails done. I bought myself some nice scented massage oil, and my beloved would rub it into my back and tummy. Another human touch can work wonders."—Amanda F.

"My husband encouraged me to go and let someone do my hair. Treating myself to a trim and style where the responsibility was in someone else's hands was nice. My husband tells me that before I'm due, I should head in to have the works—manicure, pedicure, highlights (the kind where the chemicals don't touch the skin), and whatever else I can think of, so that I'll FEEL beautiful for all the pictures he'll want to take."—Jeanie T.

"I found that keeping my hair up made me feel feminine and beautiful. My fingernails are always long and strong during pregnancy, so they were always painted, as were my toes. I often used a foot bath/massager in the later months. I took a hot shower every morning in winter and cool baths every evening in summer. I also loved getting my hair brushed."—Amelia M.

Focusing on Who You Are

While you are pregnant, it's easy to feel that *everything* is about your body. It's important to remember that you are not just about your physical body. You have talents, feelings, abilities, desires, relationships, and dreams and are so much more than just a body! Don't let your body become your complete self. Make time for the most-important part of you—that person that lives inside the pregnant attributes. Try some of these ideas for enhancing and supporting that important person.

Nurture Your Mind
- listen to music you enjoy
- read a fantastic book
- make time for a hobby
- visit a museum
- spend some time poking around the library
- take a class or lessons in something new

- make time to work on a project you've been putting off
- devote some extra time to a project at work, and do a stunning job
- take a class about something you've always wanted to learn
- do a challenging puzzle

Nurture Your Spirit

- enjoy nature
- decorate your home for the current season
- play some music on an instrument
- rent a movie you've always wanted to see
- dance in your living room
- arrange some fresh flowers
- learn a new prayer or song
- visit a favorite store, and buy yourself a present that has nothing to do with the baby
- rearrange your furniture (with some help)
- organize your photographs
- keep a journal of your dreams
- think about women you have been close to who have passed away and how they might be able to give you strength and support
- plan a trip you would like to take someday
- cook a special meal
- keep a diary
- lay on the ground and watch clouds
- learn to meditate
- walk in the grass without shoes
- organize your closet
- use the good dishes—without a special occasion
- use paper plates so there are no dishes to do
- do some charity work, or donate items to a charity

- frame some favorite photos
- learn to sew
- play a game
- write a poem or story
- visit a favorite restaurant
- surf the Internet
- sketch a picture
- build something by yourself

Nurture Your Relationships

- have a date night with your partner
- have a girls' night out with your best friends
- do something nice for someone else
- spend time with family
- have a special lunch with your mom
- get a pet (but consider if you will have time to care for it after the baby comes)
- write a letter to an old friend
- have a get-together with your siblings
- get in touch with a long-lost relative
- start a family tree
- start a pregnancy journal, or write letters to your baby
- talk to your mother or other relatives about their births and new parenting experiences

"I am a part-time opera singer, and pregnancy actually really helps your voice. So I sang like crazy! I went to networking events; I traveled. I figured, after the baby comes, I'll be really limited, better do everything now."—Liz R.

"Sometimes I got kind of sick of how everything was about my body. Throwing myself into work was a wonderful distraction for me and helped me remember that I had a brain, too."—Gail D.

Remember What Your Body Is Doing

Remind yourself occasionally of the hard work your body is doing. Think about the energy it takes for your body to not only nourish itself, but also to provide food, oxygen, and warmth for the little one inside you twenty-four hours a day. Your body is really working overtime at this nine-month project. Keep this in mind when you feel tired or cranky. Give yourself a lot of credit for what you are doing. This isn't a time in your life when you should be critical of your body or try to hold it up to some impossible standard. This is a time to revel in and enjoy the amazing things that are happening.

You have so much to plan for, so many changes to face, and so many feelings to deal with. Creating this new life takes a toll on you emotionally, as well as physically.

If you remind yourself every once in a while of these things, you'll be able to think about your body and your pregnancy in a positive and enjoyable way.

9

Beyond Sacks and Muumuus:
Plus-Size Maternity Clothes

*I*t's one thing to feel good about your body and who you are, but it's another thing entirely to feel good about the clothes you're wearing and the way they make you look. Finding and buying maternity clothes can be a challenge for any woman, but the selection becomes even smaller when you are looking for plus-sizes. It's almost as if most clothing designers think plus-size women don't need (or maybe deserve?) maternity clothes. You absolutely do. When you're pregnant, your waist is going to get bigger, even if you don't gain a lot of weight, and many regular clothes are simply not cut for a pregnant belly. You *can* find flattering maternity clothes that fit.

"I was a size 18 with my first pregnancy, and I foolishly thought I could go into any maternity store and find clothes that would fit. Wrong! In one store, the XL clothes wouldn't even go on my body."—Karen K.

"That would have to be one of the most troublesome parts of pregnancy—no clothes!"—Angie G.

"You go to Sears, and they have three tops in your size and three hundred for regular sizes. Ugh, don't get me started! Have you seen what they try and pass off as plus-size lingerie? Or bras!"—Carla R.

"I worked at Motherhood Maternity during my first pregnancy and received an employee discount, but I didn't fit in their clothes!"—Beth U.

Clothes Make the Woman

Let's face it. You're just not going to feel good about yourself if you spend your pregnancy in a giant T-shirt and sweatpants or in too-tight maternity clothes that squeeze you in all the wrong places. If you wear clothes that look good and feel good, you're going to feel better about your body and yourself. Maternity clothes aren't just sacks in which to hide yourself. They are clothes that help you show off your good features and make your growing tummy look beautiful.

Clothes are a way to express yourself and to project your self-image. This shouldn't be put on hold because you're pregnant. Rita Farro, plus-size author of *Life is Not a Dress Size: Rita Farro's Guide to Attitude, Style, and a New You*, says, "The key to dressing well during a pregnancy is to be true to yourself. If before getting pregnant you liked yourself in turtlenecks, then you should still be wearing turtlenecks. If you hated scarves, you're still gonna hate them."

If you slump around in baggy, loose clothes all the time, you'll never really see your changing shape or highlight your great legs or your gorgeous collarbone. If you wear pants that are tight in the butt or tops that pull under the shoulders, you're going to feel cranky. Wearing unattractive or ill-fitting clothing is going to affect your self-image. If you dress like you're ashamed of your body or don't care about it, that attitude will soon become part of your mind-set. But if you dress as if your body is important and you are a beautiful woman, you will soon believe you are (and other people will see that you are).

"I think wearing maternity clothes really helps to basically put up the sign 'Hey! I'm pregnant!' I bought larger regular clothes, but they never fit right. The shoulders were always too wide."—Ali S.

"I've read that a lot of women have worn sweats throughout their pregnancy. I think it makes me feel better to get up every day and dress like I did before I was pregnant."—Jill G.

Dressing for the In-between Stage

There will come a point in your pregnancy when your current clothes no longer fit, but maternity clothes just seem like huge tents. By the time you're in your second or third month of pregnancy, you may start to feel as if you need to do something about your wardrobe, but you have no idea what. It seems ridiculous to go out and buy clothes in a larger size that aren't going to fit through the end of your pregnancy, and you can't imagine wearing giant maternity clothes yet.

There are solutions for this no man's (or more correctly, woman's) land. First, examine your current wardrobe. You probably have some loose sweaters and dresses that you can continue to use. Pants with elastic waists or spandex may last you a while longer. This is also a good time to do a closet sweep. If it doesn't fit now, it's not going to fit for at least a couple months after the baby comes, so you might as well get it out of sight and out of mind. Push things to the back of the closet or put them away in another room. You're not supposed to be able to fit into those things anymore—you're pregnant!

Think about ways to make other clothing last. Buy waistband expanders and bra extenders. Waistband expanders attach to the buttons on your skirts or pants and add a piece of elastic and some space so you can continue wearing these items a while longer. There is also a new product called a Bella Band (which comes in plus-size). This is a very wide elastic belt that will slip over the waistband of pants or skirts, holding them in place, even if you can't close them. Bra extenders attach to the hooks and eyes of your bras and add extra inches to the band of the bra.

You can find waistband expanders online at: *store.babycenter.com/product/clothing/moms_essentials/maternity/5176* or *www.kidsurplus.com/maternity.html*. They are also often available in maternity stores. Find Bella Band at *www.bellaband.com*. Bra extenders can be found at sewing stores or maternity stores.

"I used a rubber-band hair tie to extend my jeans. I looped it through the buttonhole and fastened it around my button. This gave me the extra inches I needed to be comfortable without the expense of buying extenders."—Vanessa R.

Rita Farro suggests moving into maternity clothes right away. "Enjoy a few weeks of people saying 'That top is way too big on you.'" Maternity clothes will definitely be comfortable at this stage of the game, and you'll have a lot of fun wearing your new items.

Choosing Not to Buy Maternity Clothes

Plus-Size maternity clothes can be hard to find. It can be difficult to find something in your size, let alone something that fits your budget and your fashion sense. And if none of the stores near you carry plus-sizes, your only choice may be ordering online, which some women prefer not to do. Wearing larger-size regular clothing not only expands your wardrobe, it offers you more-attractive and affordable choices. Nothing says you have to wear maternity clothes if you don't want to. Many women buy some maternity clothes and some regular-size clothes. Nonmaternity tops often end up looking too short in the front during the last trimester, but some styles may work for you. Consider new travel knits, which are stretchy and comfortable, as well as trapeze or baby-doll-style tops, legging-style pants, and loose-fitting dresses. Elastic is your friend, and pants and skirts with elastic waists will work as long as you buy them large enough.

Buy nonmaternity clothing that is one or two sizes larger than what you normally wear. These companies have stores and Web sites that can offer some choices of regular plus-size clothing that may work for you during pregnancy:

- Catherine's Plus Sizes (*www.catherines.com*)
- Coldwater Creek (*www.coldwatercreek.com*)
- Fashion Bug (*www.fashionbug.com*)
- Lane Bryant (*www.lanebryant.com*)
- Igigi (*www.igigi.com*)
- Torrid (*www.torrid.com*)

The following do not have actual stores, but have Web sites:

- Draper's & Damon's (*www.drapers.com*)
- JMS: Just My Size (*www.justmysize.com*)
- Junonia (*www.junonia.com*)
- Making It Big (*www.makingitbigonline.com*)
- Plus Woman (*www.pluswoman.com*). This site will custom make clothes to fit your body
- QVC (*www.qvc.com*)
- Silhouettes (*www.Silhouettes.com*)
- Ulla Popken (*www.ullapopken.com*)
- Zaftique (*www.zaftique.com*)

Rita Farro says, "Most stores that cater to plus-sizes emphasize separates, and that can work in our favor during pregnancy. Many styles are meant to be worn loosely, not tucked in. When it comes to tops, you'll want to choose nonmaternity styles that are fuller, meant to be worn out. Maybe tunic length, maybe gathered on a front yoke, etc.

Depending on the cut of the garment, you may not even have to buy a bigger size top, just a different, fuller style."

"I did buy regular clothes—one size up. Wal-Mart has a good selection of plus-size clothes."—Angie G.

"I found it cheaper to buy clothes in larger sizes. I looked for baby-doll-style clothes and bought them a size bigger."—Lisa B.

"I got a couple of skirts with elastic waistbands. I think I bought two sizes larger."—Becky A.

"I think it's a waste of money to buy larger clothes that aren't maternity. They just don't fit the same. In maternity clothing, you find styles that leave room in the belly, but don't make you look like a linebacker at the same time."—Jill G.

"With my first pregnancy I wore a 22/24. So I would go to Lane Bryant and buy a 26/28 to wear during the pregnancy."—Beth U.

"I think plus-size moms without a lot of money, (I know I didn't have a lot) should try and find larger regular clothing cheaply at consignment thrift shops and garage sales, and only get things like undergarments at stores like Lane Bryant (because you don't want to wear secondhand underwear!)"—DeAnn R.

"I wore a lot of my husband's shirts and shorts."—Deb P.

If you can't find a maternity coat, or don't want to buy a coat you won't be able to use again, consider a poncho or cape. You might also be able to get away with your own coats by wearing them unbuttoned.

What Size to Buy

When buying maternity clothes, you should generally buy the same size you wore before your pregnancy. Practically speaking, this may not always work. Consider clothes up one size and down one size if you are having problems finding things that fit. Everyone's body changes in different ways, and you might find your butt expands while your tummy doesn't go anywhere, or that your thighs have decided to be pregnant, too. Pay special attention to the fit in the chest and hip area. These are likely to expand, and if something just fits in those areas now, you won't have room if your body changes. Manufacturers who make regular-size clothing sometimes make the mistake of oversizing armholes or length when they modify designs to make plus-size items, so don't assume the manufacturer will design appropriately. Remember that manufacturers vary widely. What is an XL in one store might be a size 14 in another.

When you try on maternity clothes, it helps to use the store's baby pillow. This is a small pillow that is shaped to replicate how your belly will grow later in your pregnancy. If the store doesn't have one, grasp the top or pants material covering your belly, and pull it out to see how it will look with a baby growing underneath it, or stuff another balled-up shirt underneath.

Clothes that are Flattering and Comfortable

Not all maternity clothes are created equal. Some are clearly cut for thin women with basketball stomachs, while others are more flattering for plus-size women. Pay careful attention to the material and how it feels against your skin. Your body is going to be rubbing against clothing in ways you never imagined. If something feels scratchy or unyielding now, it's sure to be something you won't want to wear as you get bigger.

Pants that have exposed elastic on the waistbands can become uncomfortable as the elastic cuts into your tummy. You may also find that as your pregnancy progresses, you turn into a human furnace and only natural, breathable fibers will feel comfortable.

Barbara Brickner, plus-size model and owner of plus-size maternity company BB Maternity says, "Quality is the hardest thing to find for the plus and pregnant woman. You may find a cute style in a top, but it may only last a couple of washes. The first thing to look for is the content of the fabric. If it is 100 percent cotton with no lycra at all, you know that this garment will shrink up in length. Make sure that you know your fabric before you purchase anything on the expensive side. If the garment is a bit short, know that as your belly grows, your garment will shorten as well. It is vital that you purchase items that are longer in the front than in the back—by at least an inch if not two. I would say in almost every case, that maternity wear should have some sort of stretch to it. Lycra is great with cotton and matte jersey polyester is also great. Anything with a bit of lycra blend is going to form to your body and stretch with you."

Remember that you don't have to hide your belly. Just look at all the photos of pregnant movie stars walking around wearing tight tops or bare midriffs. Baby bumps are definitely in. But it's all a matter of individual taste and preference. If you're comfortable in it and think it looks good, wear it.

Some women find that the best way to stay comfortable during pregnancy is to have some of their regular clothes altered to become maternity clothes. This way you know the item feels good and looks good. See later in the chapter for information about sewing and altering.

"I think nice, loose sweaters look best on pregnant women in cool weather and sleeveless tunics in the summer."—Ali S.

"I hated the jeans and pants with the belly section. I thought those were very uncomfortable. I thought the most-flattering clothes were tunic/long tops over pants made of stretchy knits—not too tight or too stretchy. Dresses were flattering."—Michelle C.

"My favorite shirts when I got to the final months were swing-style tops with an empire waist and a tie in the back. They were very comfortable and could be casual or dressed up with accessories."—Becky A.

"Don't be afraid to wear formfitting tops. They're much more flattering. And no stirrup or tight legged pants—very unattractive! Wide leg or boot-cut pull the eyes down."—Amelia M.

Wardrobe Pieces You Need

The types of clothes you need depend on your career and lifestyle. But most women find they need at the very minimum:

- at least one dress (more if you need them for work)
- one or two skirts
- four pairs of pants
- six tops
- two coordinated pants and tops outfits
- two sweaters or sweatshirts
- three maternity bras
- eight maternity panties (or larger-size regular panties)
- two pairs of maternity hose or larger-size hose (more if you have to wear them to work)
- A coat to suit your climate

If you wear suits to work, purchase two or three maternity suits and several dresses. You may be able to wear prepregnancy blouses under your suits if you don't button them all the way down (or if you wear pullover tops and just let them ride up on your tummy) and if you keep the suit jacket buttoned. There aren't many maternity sleepwear items available that are not nursing nightgowns, so your best bet is to wear something you have or go find something big and cheap that you won't mind tossing when the pregnancy is over.

Evening wear can be especially difficult during a plus-size pregnancy. Brickner says, "I love the idea of the poncho for plus women and evening wear. You can pair a sheer poncho over a tank with a fabulous pair of black pants and a wedge heel and amazing jewelry." She also recommends a wrap dress paired with jewelry for evening wear and points out that both ponchos and wrap dresses are versatile enough to be dressed down for daytime and dressed up for evening wear and can become essential wardrobe pieces.

Rita Farro says, "Maybe there is no 'basic wardrobe' for a pregnant woman. Whatever kind of clothes you wore in your before-pregnancy life—whether it's blue jeans or business suits—you should best figure out a way to make those clothes work during pregnancy. That said, every pregnant woman should have black knit pants and a long, black skirt. The style, accessorizing, and change of mood can happen on top—bringing the focus up to your face."

"Pants are the hardest thing to find. Most of them are either way too big or way too small."—Ali S.

"Ponchos are in, and while I don't like them for myself, I think they're really flattering on plus-size women."—Jill G.

"My worst complaint is paneled pants—uncomfortable and impossible for a plus-size woman to hide with tops that aren't long enough."—Cheryl H.

Accessorize Your Outfits

If you're buying a limited number of clothes, you will easily grow tired of them unless you find ways to dress them up. Buying scarves, jewelry, and wraps will help your clothes feel a little bit different every time you wear them. And any accessories you buy during pregnancy can be used postpregnancy, so it's not wasted money.

If you think scarves might work for you, consider buying a book to help you find new and different ways to tie them. There are many books that are out of print and available used on Amazon.com, or you can purchase *Sensational Scarfs: 44 Great Ways to Turn a Scarf into a Fabulous Fashion Look* by Carol Straley.

Rita Farro says that wearing solid bottoms and patterned tops will give you the most bang for your buck. "This is magical. If you do it right, every top you have will coordinate with every bottom, multiplying your choices."

Where to Buy Maternity Clothes

Most maternity stores do not carry true plus sizes. Many carry an XL size, and some carry sizes 18 to 20 in limited amounts. Brickner says, "It seems very strange to me that the maternity world does not want to cater to the plus woman. When I first started my company, I called a clothing representative in a major market for maternity. She actually laughed when I explained that I wanted to bring maternity clothes to the plus market in a dignified manner! I was appalled. I have learned that the maternity world of fashion usually runs 5-7 years behind the normal fashion trends. I can't explain it, but I think this must be the only explanation for NOT carrying plus on the current maternity label leaders."

Instead of dragging yourself around to all the local maternity stores, sit down with the phone book first, and call and ask them the sizes they carry. Don't just ask if they carry plus sizes—ask them specifically to name the sizes they have in stock. Don't be surprised to find them stuffed on a rack at the back of the store, either. When you go, ask where the plus sizes are so you don't spend time fruitlessly flipping through every rack only to find that most things end with a size L. Large retailers such as J.C. Penney, Kmart, Wal-Mart, Sears, Target, Fashion Bug, and Motherhood Maternity frequently carry plus-size maternity clothes.

Remember to try consignment stores, but call them first to find out if they have any maternity clothes in your size. The selection at these stores can be quite wide if you hit the right one. You may also be able to leave your name and number with the store and have them call you if they receive any stock in your size.

Shopping online is an excellent way to find plus-size maternity clothes, however the downside is that you can't try on items before purchasing. When shopping online, always check to see if the site has a size chart so that you can get a sense of how the sizes run.

Plus-Size Maternity Clothing Stores and Sites
- Fashion Bug, *www.fashionbug.com*
- J.C. Penney, *www.jcpenney.com*. J.C. Penney has plus sizes on its Web site and also publishes a maternity catalog that includes plus sizes. If you have a store near you, you can have your order sent to the store and pick it up there, saving on shipping costs.
- Motherhood Maternity, *www.motherhood.com*
- BB Maternity, *www.bbmaternity.com*. This site is a wholesaler, but includes a list of stores where you can find their clothes.
- Due Maternity, *www.duematernity.com*. This company sells clothes online and also has boutiques in various areas.

Plus-Size Maternity Web sites
- Plus Mom Maternity, *www.plusmommaternity.com*
- Jake and Me, *www.jakeandme.com*
- Baby Becoming Maternity, *www.babybecoming.com*
- Maternity 4 Less, *www.maternity4less.com*
- Pickles & Ice Cream, *www.plusmaternity.com*
- imaternity, *www.imaternity.com*
- QVC, *www.qvc.com*. Search for maternity on its site. QVC carries the Mommy & Co. label, which comes in plus sizes.
- Maternity Clothing Fashions, *www.maternity-clothing-fashions.com*
- Mom's Maternity, *www.momsmaternity.com*

Another good choice online is eBay, *www.ebay.com*. You may even be able to buy an entire wardrobe in one purchase. When using eBay, check the seller's rating, and types of payment accepted, and make sure you understand shipping costs before purchase. You can trade and swap plus-size maternity clothes at OPSS, OMOMs and Big Moms Trading Arena, *www.network54.com/Forum/goto?forumid=14843*.

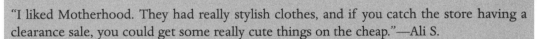

"The best place to buy plus-size maternity clothes would be Kmart for me."—Lisa B.

"I liked Motherhood. They had really stylish clothes, and if you catch the store having a clearance sale, you could get some really cute things on the cheap."—Ali S.

"I think that for a plus-size woman larger than a size 20, your luck runs out with most stores. Motherhood Maternity has a decent selection of clothing, but it's depressing because the clothing for smaller women is much cuter. Other places I've looked, including online, seem to think that drape clothing is where it's at. No offense to them, but they need to learn that pregnant women are not sixty years old! I do think it would be nice if Motherhood wouldn't assume that pregnant women who are overweight are also six feet tall."—Jill G.

"I searched the online plus sites and found them atrocious! I wanted style and a few sexier looks to wear out with my husband, but they had these short-sleeve tents and caftanlike tops and dresses that no one should even have to look at. I wanted something with a bit of shape to it and some plunge with length."—Cheryl H.

"Everything was purchased online at Pickles & Ice Cream. The lady who runs the site is very helpful in picking out clothes for you."—Jennifer H.

"My online favorites were Motherhood, Jake and Me, and Baby Becoming."—Margie P.

"If I were to become pregnant now—bite your tongue!—I'd try eBay first. I did well at consignment stores in upscale areas."—Michelle C.

"Other Mothers is one of my favorite places to shop because women take their old clothes there for store credit on baby clothes, and they have a wide assortment of sizes."—Ali S.

If you sew, *http://patternsthatfityou.com/Maternity.htm* offers a book that explains how to convert regular patterns into maternity clothes. Plus-size maternity is especially mentioned. Another site, *www.simplicity.com*, offers plus-size maternity sewing patterns, and *www.isewplus.com* is a site run by a woman who sews custom-made plus-size maternity clothing.

Plus-Size style expert Farro remembers helping her niece modify a pair of regular pants into maternity pants. "We opened up the side seam (on both sides), from the waistband down, about six inches. Then we used two safety pins to attach a six-inch piece of one-inch-wide black elastic on each side. As she got bigger, she would simply adjust the safety pin. She always wore these pants with a long tunic top. And, she was lucky enough to have black underpants."

"I had some [plus-size maternity clothes] designed for me, and I felt great! I now lend them out to other plus-size mothers. I felt really special as maternity clothes emphasize the bump and take away the flab."—Rachel G.

"I was very lucky that my mother sews. We had to get the largest size pattern [for maternity clothes] and alter them to fit."—Vanessa R.

Undergarments

Maternity bras and panties are available at *www.biggerbras.com*. You may find that buying a bigger size regular panty and wearing it under your belly is a comfortable option. If you buy a maternity bra, buy your regular size. If you are shopping for a larger-size regular bra, look for something up one band and cup size. Cotton bras may be the most comfortable. (For information about nursing bras, see Chapter 15.)

J.C. Penney and Baby Becoming carry plus-size maternity hose. Some women find that buying larger regular hose works well; *www.justmysize.com* carries plus-size hose.

Belly-support garments can be found at *www.growinglife.com*. These elastic belts are worn underneath your tummy and help provide back support in the last trimester.

Specialty Items and Sizes

If you're looking for a gown or wedding gown, *www.maternity-clothing-fashions.com* has a nice selection. If you have to be in a wedding as a bridesmaid during your pregnancy, tell the bride what size you normally wear and let her know about your pregnancy as soon as possible. It

"I would not have made it without my support garment. It was ugly and looked like a truss or something, but I had terrible groin pain during my pregnancy. I went to a medical supply store and bought this contraption that was a wide elastic band that went under my belly and then had a crisscross in the back and shoulder straps. It really helped take the pressure off my groin muscles. It was ugly as sin, and sometimes it peeked out of the collar of my top, which I hated."—Brenda M.

"I had debilitating back pain in one of my pregnancies. [A belly support garment] helped a lot, but you can get so used to it that your back muscles can become weaker and more susceptible to injury. Use all of them with caution."—Amelia M.

"I got a pregnancy girdle from J.C. Penney. It was ugly as hell, but it helped with the pressure and strain. I had to buy bras two different times while pregnant. Go to a good store, and be measured. There is nothing worse than being uncomfortable due to an ill-fitting bra!"—Becky A.

"I didn't wear any pantyhose at all while pregnant because I couldn't find any reasonably priced and comfortable. Finding panties was the absolute worst. All of the maternity panties were expensive and made of material that was itchy and caused a rash."—Michelle C.

"Motherhood had the best underwear. As far as hose was concerned, I shopped at Catherine's and bought a larger size without control top."—Carla R.

"Finding big undies that could expand with my belly was a bit of a problem."—Sharon L.

"I started out with enormous breasts—very long and pendulous. Bras started hurting immediately because the top of my stomach popped so early. The underwire bras push down on my stomach, and the soft cup bras pinch, and sadly, I'm just too huge to go without. So I'm looking for solutions now."—Liz O.

"We sold a lot of [belly support garments when I was] working at Motherhood Maternity, and people swore by them."—Beth U.

"I tried [a belly support garment] by Baby Becoming, and I did like it and found it useful, but it was a hassle going to the bathroom."—Julie M.

may impact what she can choose from, although if the gowns she selects come in plus sizes, they can usually be altered to be wearable during pregnancy.

If you need scrubs, try *www.sassyscrubs.com* and *www.scrubs-r-us.com*. Bathing suits can be found at *www.plusmaternity.com* or *www.jcpenney.com*. Both stores also carry maternity plus-size business suits, and *www.babybecoming.com* has some maternity plus-size coats.

You can find tall plus sizes at *www.jakeandme.com*, and *www.maternity-clothing-fashions.com* carries plus-size petites. If you need larger-size plus sizes, *www.jakeandme.com*, *www.plusmaternity.com*, and *www.babybecoming.com* carry sizes above 3x.

"I did buy courtroom-appropriate dresses and pants outfits (I was a practicing attorney) at Motherhood Maternity and Catherine's."—Carla R.

"I found a very nice maternity suit in the J.C. Penney catalog. The skirt had a sleeveless top (not meant to be seen) attached to it so it didn't bind at the waist at all. It was a neutral beige, and it went with a lot of blouses."—Lee T.

"I got petites at Motherhood Maternity."—Melissa S.

"I am also tall, but most plus-size maternity clothing seemed to be targeted for tall people. I often wondered what a five-foot-two-inch gal would do."—Margie P.

Shoes

Although you normally don't think of your feet as being affected by pregnancy, feet can grow a size, become wider, or just be puffier during pregnancy (not to mention achier). If you must be on your feet at work, investing in some good, comfortable shoes will be an expense you won't regret. Easy Spirit (*www.easyspirit.com*) makes a wide variety of comfortable and attractive shoes with sizes up to 12 and widths up to double wide.

If you wear heels, consider switching to a lower or squarer heel for additional stability. You might also want to avoid pointy toes and opt for a wider-cut shoe. For casual wear, sneakers are a great choice, as are slides.

"I splurged and got some really comfortable Adidas running shoes. The high price was really worth it because my swollen feet had support and room to grow."—Ali S.

"Wear comfortable shoes, no matter where you're going. I grew a full shoe size during pregnancy."—Liz R.

"Wear shoes with low, wide heels—not completely flat."—Carla R.

"My feet got wider during pregnancy. I went from wearing a 9 to wearing a 9 wide—and the bad news is they didn't shrink back after pregnancy."—Linda O.

"My feet were frequently swollen, so I stopped wearing regular shoes and wore flip-flops absolutely everywhere."—Beth U.

10

Dealing with Self-Esteem and Stress

*S*elf-esteem is one of the biggest issues facing plus-size women. Our shape is not celebrated or accepted by society, and we often come to think of ourselves as second-class citizens. Being pregnant and plus size can be a downer when people look at you askance, can't tell that you're pregnant, or say tactless things. Self-esteem issues are buried deep within us—we can't blame it all on other people. Self-esteem has to do with emotional health. And pregnancy is THE time in your life to focus on health. Finding ways to increase and improve your self-esteem will make you happier, more comfortable, and better prepared to be a mom.

Self-Esteem

If you had self-esteem issues before you were pregnant, you may find one of two things happen. Some women feel supremely self-confident and positive about their plus-size bodies during pregnancy because they feel as if their body is doing something worthwhile and important. Other women find that they feel even worse about themselves, certain that people are whispering about their size and uncomfortable that their body is even more on display than ever before. If you're having self-esteem problems, it can take some work, but you can feel positive about yourself.

"Self-esteem is a tricky matter that so many people, especially heavy people, struggle with," says Dr. Merry McVey-Noble, plus-size cognitive behavioral psychologist at the Bio-Behavioral Institute and professor of psychology at Hofstra University. "Who you are as a person has little to do with your body. It's your spirit, your intellect, your kindness, your humor, and all of the intangibles that make you unique. If you base your self-esteem on your body, whoever you are, you will have a very unstable sense of it because our bodies change all the time. Really work to maintain your sense of who you are and you will be able to weather any physical changes that occur. Remember, you want to treat yourself with esteem and respect because you want your child to see you that way and to grow up feeling self-esteem and respect."

Finding self-esteem is about more than just accepting your body. Accepting your body for what it is and learning to love it is an important step, but self-esteem is about appreciating and respecting your entire self. Many women who are plus-sized hate not only their bodies, but themselves. They believe that there is something fundamentally wrong or flawed with their personalities or entire being that allows them to be the size they are. Overcoming this can be painful and difficult. But having good self-esteem is important, because you are now going to be a role model for a little person whom you want to have a healthy self-esteem.

To build your self-esteem, try these tips:

Notice the good
Too often we're too busy tearing ourselves down to notice what is good. Really take the time to think about the things you are exceptional at,

and put a spotlight on your good qualities as you did in chapter 1. The more you think about your positive qualities, the more proud of them you will be. Stop sweeping these attributes under the carpet.

Make more room for success

Make time to do the things you are good at and that give you pleasure and a feeling of satisfaction. It's too easy to become so busy that you don't have time for things which might seem nonessential, but really are essential in making you happy.

Choose happiness

Deliberately make choices in your life that allow you to feel happy. Choose to look at the positives instead of harping on the negatives in your life and about yourself. It's OK to work on changing things that make you unhappy, but it's not OK to dwell on them.

Be with positive people

Surround yourself with people who make you feel good about yourself—this includes family, friends, and health-care providers. If you see a smiling face everywhere you look, you will begin to feel good about yourself.

Reward yourself

Do good things for yourself simply because you deserve it. No one else in your life is going to give you a gold star, so do it for yourself.

Set goals for yourself and meet them

It can be hard to begin to see yourself in a positive light if you aren't happy with who you are or what you've been doing. Setting some goals that are within reach, and then going after them, can give you an immediate self-esteem boost. You'll know not only that you accomplished a goal, but also that you had the stamina, self-belief, and oomph to do it. It doesn't matter if these goals have to do with your job, your relationships, or things in your everyday life. Specifically setting goals, and then meeting them, creates a pattern of positive living that will make you feel good about yourself.

"Men find pregnant women sexy, so don't feel ashamed because you're bigger. Feel empowered and sexy. Walk tall, and shake what your mother gave you."—Ali S.

"I felt like everyone was looking at me. It seemed that all I ever saw were glowing pregnant women. Every place I looked, there were women who, other than the small basketball under their shirt, didn't even look pregnant. I recall hating how I looked. Passing a mirrored wall in the mall could make me cry. I felt I looked terrible."—Michelle C.

"Look in the mirror naked every day. I don't know, it just seems if you can look at yourself with no problems that way, then it doesn't feel so bad that everyone is looking at you with your clothes on."—Shannan E.

"My best girlfriend once had a poster up in college that has always stayed with me. It read, 'No one can make you feel inferior without your consent.' Trouble is, I tend to consent when at my lowest ebb in morale! Pregnancy is hard because, although I am so blessed with this miracle inside me growing, I don't like the feeling of being so heavy. I have to keep looking at my children to remind myself that this is temporary and all worth it. My vanity has taken a beating to be sure. But my husband and my children have helped me figure out that life is more than what I look like right now. I know that I need to be responsible for how I feel."—Cheryl H.

Getting Respect

To get respect from others, you must first have respect for yourself. This means believing that you are a worthwhile person who deserves kindness, love, and a happy life. Once you begin to believe you deserve respect, you must start acting like it. If you put yourself down, degrade yourself, or act in a way that shows disrespect for your body and yourself, it is a signal to other people that they can treat you the same way. But if you carry yourself as a woman who is important and who deserves to be treated well, then others will also begin to see you in this way.

Dr. McVey-Noble points out that part of getting respect is calling out those who do not offer it to you. "Don't tolerate people whose behavior is degrading or condescending. Address them immediately and effectively."

Addressing unkind words or attitudes can be difficult, particularly if you don't feel self-confident. You can remove yourself from the situation so you don't have to deal with the problem. You can ignore the words or behavior that bothers you. You can also choose to directly tell the person that what they've done or said has hurt your feelings. Many women interviewed for this book reported feeling a lack of respect in many aspects of their lives—from coworkers, health-care professionals, strangers, store clerks, and even their spouses.

There will always be unkind or ignorant people who say or do rude things. While you can affect how those closest to you treat you, you can't change the acts of strangers. But you can change who you are so that you are secure in your love and respect for yourself, and then are able to ignore or rise above ignorance.

"Overall, I think it's helpful to simply adopt an attitude that no one else's opinion matters. Because you will find yourself in the face of women who don't gain a lot of weight and who seem to radiate beauty. And you will have critics. But let them worry about themselves. You just worry about you and your baby."—Michelle C.

Invisible Pregnancy Syndrome

You know you're pregnant, your partner and family and friends know your pregnant, but you might be worried that other people aren't able to tell. In fact, this can be one of the most upsetting parts of a plus-size pregnancy. You are so elated and excited, yet feel people can't see that you're actually pregnant. You're getting bigger every day, but strangers just give you those dismissive or disgusted looks they reserve for heavy people. They don't have a clue that you're pregnant and don't usually walk around with a tummy this big.

Every pregnancy goes through the invisible stage. Even the skinniest of the skinny women who develop the cute basketball bellies go through periods where they are just thicker and bloated instead of adorably pregnant. (Imagine their horror when people think they've put on some weight instead of knowing they are pregnant.) The problem can be especially pronounced when people are used to seeing you in clothing that is not formfitting. Your pregnancy may not be completely obvious (even though when you look in a mirror, it seems pretty clear to you). Sometimes people develop a blind spot. They notice a woman is plus-sized and then just assume that bulge around her middle is the result of too many ice-cream sundaes.

So how do you deal with invisible pregnancy syndrome? First, it's important to recognize and honor your pregnancy in your daily life so you're not relying on other people to provide the sense of joy you need in pregnancy. (See Chapter 12 for more information.) Do things that affirm your pregnancy, like shopping for baby clothes, decorating the nursery, thinking over baby names, registering for your shower, and so on. Taking active steps in your life that imprint the fact of your pregnancy will help you feel better about the fact that not everyone can obviously see what's happening inside your uterus.

Choosing the right clothes can help make your pregnancy more obvious. Some styles of tops show off your belly more than others. If you want people to be able to tell you're pregnant, try on several styles to see what emphasizes your belly. (Chapter 9 has more information about this.)

Telling people that you are pregnant can make you feel better and put them at ease. Many women interviewed for this book described a need to tell acquaintances and strangers, finding a way to work it into conversation. Doing this can take the guessing out of the situation and make you feel more comfortable. If you want word to spread in your workplace, casually mentioning your good news to the biggest gossip is an easy way to get the news out. Some women report choosing clothing that announces their pregnancy (with storks or "baby on board" designs), so the guesswork is eliminated.

The best way to deal with invisible pregnancy syndrome is to just accept that the entire world may not be able to see your happy news right now, but that before your baby is born, it will become obvious. There are not many eight- or nine-month pregnant women walking around who are not recognizably pregnant. And for now, the most important people in your life know and are celebrating your joy with you.

Tactful ways to mention your pregnancy:

- You don't mind if I sit down, do you? I'm five months pregnant and get so tired sometimes.

- I'm sorry to be in a hurry, but I've got to get to my OB appointment.

- I'm trying to get all of these things done before my baby is born.

- That's a beautiful baby. I'm due in September.

- Would you like a piece of gum? I'm pregnant, and it seems to help with my nausea.

- Yes, I do have an awful cold, but I'm expecting, and my doctor won't let me take anything for it

"It's hard to tell I'm pregnant until about the fifth month. I just look fatter. I try to wear bigger clothes (nonconforming) until I have that nice, round belly."—Amelia M.

"I had that with the first pregnancy. It was terrible. I couldn't wear my own clothes as soon as nine weeks. No kidding. I couldn't wear them. But I had no discernible belly, and it remained this way until I was roughly six months or so. It was awful. I mostly just didn't make eye contact with people or made a point of saying I was pregnant—which was probably not the way to handle it."—Michelle C.

"Lay your hands on top of the swell; that is an unmistakable sign. You don't see just anyone doing that!"—Ali S.

"YES! This was a huge issue. It's like you have the hassles of pregnancy and you don't get public credit for them! People would look at me, and I could see them evaluating, 'Is she pregnant, fat, or both?' So I'd make it easier for them by subtly mentioning that I WAS pregnant by saying 'Nice to meet you! Would you mind if we sat down? I can really feel the baby kicking.' That would get us over the hurdle."—Liz R.

"I am just starting my third trimester, and only now am I starting to show. This is the part I have hated most about pregnancy because I feel pregnant and close family and friends notice, but I just don't have that cute baby belly!"—Jennifer N.

"I was walking through the mall with my pregnant belly displayed for the entire world to see. This guy actually walked by me and said in passing that someone needed to call 1-800-Jenny. I felt horrible for days."—Richelle H.

"When I was about five months pregnant with my first child, one of my GED students found out I was pregnant from another student and said, 'Oh, I didn't know you were pregnant. I just thought you were round and fat.' That really hurt me. I was so proud of the little creature growing in me. I wanted everyone to know, but it was then that I realized that I just looked fat to most everyone. Even though I could see the difference—see my stomach taking the pregnancy shape—no one else could. In fact, I don't believe people were brave enough to mention my pregnancy until I was about seven months or so."—Dana C.

"Through my first two pregnancies, unless I was wearing maternity clothes, no one would guess I was pregnant. My last pregnancy, I really looked pregnant. However at seven-plus months, I was talking at work about my pregnancy (while wearing a smocked top covering my huge pregnant belly) and a thin coworker said, 'Oh, are you pregnant?'"—Margie P.

Managing Stress

Pregnancy is a stressful time. Even though it's a time filled with joy, you're undergoing a major life change, one that will affect you for years and years to come. In addition, you have a medical condition that has to be constantly monitored—even if your pregnancy is completely normal—and this can make you anxious. Many women worry about the baby and about their health, as well. And for plus-size women, that worry is intensified because there are some heightened risks for both you and your baby.

It can be easy to let all these risks and tests and constant monitoring get to you. You could spend your entire day recalculating your risk of neural-tube defects or preeclampsia. Worrying about it isn't going to help, though, and it's only going to make you feel worse, both physically and emotionally.

The best way to deal with your worries is to get informed. Read everything you can, and ask your health-care providers questions. If you don't, you may be worrying about something that isn't even a possibility for you. Get your facts, and take a hard look at them. Understand exactly what the risks mean in terms of real life, real people, and real possibilities. Then find out what you can do to reduce your risks. This may mean taking your prenatal vitamin, changing your diet, going for certain tests, or other steps recommended by your health-care provider. Once you've done all you can do to reduce your risks, you have to focus on finding inner peace. This doesn't mean push all concerns to the side, but it does mean finding a way to live with them without it affecting your daily life. There are lots of ways to cope with this kind of stress—prayer, keeping a journal, talking to friends, meditation, distraction, and planned positive thinking.

"I was very worried. I was very worried I would die. I think I knew my son would be OK. I had a feeling. But I was so worried, I could hardly talk about it without getting upset. I wrote long letters to my mother and my husband and one to my son to be read in the event of my death. I also got a temporary term life insurance on myself so my husband would be OK. Morbid maybe, but I was worried."—Julie M.

"I worried when I read typical pregnancy books that tell you all the terrible, bad things that can happen when you're overweight and pregnant. Once I talked to my OB and he told me to stop reading, I relaxed. I can't believe how much is written about being overweight when there are so many worse things you can be when pregnant, like a drug addict, an alcoholic, the list can go on and on. I mean everything is the same on the inside no matter what your size. There are certain things that may be different for us, like ultrasounds, but I think when you're overweight, you deal with certain everyday things as well, you know what they are, and you handle them."—Jennifer H.

"During my first pregnancy, I worried incessantly that my baby would have problems because of my size or that I wouldn't be athletic enough to deliver a baby."—Margie P.

"Try your hardest to focus on the baby and the wonderful, miraculous thing your body is doing by creating a whole new life—a new little body—where there was nothing before."
—Carla R.

11

Stuff that Holds You Up (Beyond A Good Bra):

Finding Support

O ne of the best ways to feel good about yourself and stay positive is to talk to other people. They say it takes a village to raise a child, well, it takes a village to get you through a pregnancy, too. Getting support and encouragement from family, friends, and people in similar situations can improve your state of mind and provide reassurance. Talking through your concerns and worries helps you exorcise them, and your partner, family, and friends may be able to give you helpful suggestions or perspectives that will make you feel better about things. Relying on your community of loved ones is essential during pregnancy because you may be feeling vulnerable, scared, nervous, or uncomfortable. Let the people you love help lift you up and keep you positive.

Accepting that You Need Support
If you are a woman who finds it difficult to admit you need help, this is one time in your life when you should look for a way to knock down that barrier. Even if you are independent and self-confident, pregnancy

and new motherhood is a time when you're dealing with more than you're used to. Expressing your fears, worries, thoughts, and joy to others will help you work through them and find solutions and acceptance.

Sometimes women are reluctant to seek support out of a fear that others will affirm their negative thoughts. You can trust those that are closest to you, and they really can help you feel good about yourself and positive about your pregnancy.

It can be hard to get out the words to express what you're worried or upset about, especially when it is something as taboo as weight. Plus-size psychologist and professor Dr. Merry McVey-Noble offers these suggestions for talking about your anxieties. "First identify exactly what it is that you fear. If you can put words to it, you will automatically be closer to mastering it. Write about it to yourself and as you do so, you will sort it out and then be able to express it to others. If it seems embarrassing, imagine the conversation first, rehearse it (but not too much), and then just say it. However you say it, it will be better than keeping it in. In saying things to others, we sometimes hear our own voices and realize that our fears are not as bad as we thought they were. If they are as bad as we imagined, at least we've shared the burden."

"You need to talk about it. Don't stop talking—the more insecure you feel, the more you should be willing to put it out there."—Liz O.

"Pregnancy in and of itself opens the floodgates of vulnerability."—Cheryl H.

Your Spouse or Partner

Your spouse or partner should be the front line of support for you. You're going to be parents together. Your spouse is the one person who is (almost!) as involved in the pregnancy as you are, so you should rely on him to help you through it. Not only should you open up to him about your feelings, you should ask him to help you when you need it. There is no reason to think you have to do this all by yourself.

Some women have difficulty turning to their partners for help or emotional support, particularly when it comes to something that involves their weight. Many larger women feel embarrassed about their size and can't find a way to talk to their spouses about the way their changing bodies make them feel. Some women are afraid that if they call attention to their size, their spouse will no longer love them or find them desirable. Your partner isn't blind. He knows what you look like, and he loves your shape. Pregnancy won't change that. In fact, many men are even more attracted to their wives during pregnancy.

Dr. McVey-Noble recommends that you talk to your spouse about your feelings regarding your body. "Sometimes we find that the parts of ourselves that we loathe the most, they love the most. Allow him to model acceptance, and don't turn away, even if you're uncomfortable. Apparently, in loving you, he's connected with something in you that is great and wonderful, maybe something you don't/can't see. Try taking his perspective for a moment. See yourself as he sees you. It's generally a lot more flattering than the way we look at ourselves. Then allow yourself to be the person your spouse is in love with."

The baby belongs to him too, and its growth is an exciting thing for him to see. Sharing your feelings about the pregnancy and its effect on your body can clue him into how you're feeling and help him understand what you need from him. One of the keys to having a good relationship with your spouse during your pregnancy is to learn to love your own body. It is difficult to accept someone else's love if you can't love yourself.

Pregnancy not only changes your body, it changes your emotions. There is a lot going on inside you, both physically and emotionally, and there is no way your spouse can understand how you're feeling or what you're thinking unless you tell him. Sometimes women think it should be obvious how they are feeling. Well, to another woman, maybe it is, but to a man who has no idea what it's like to be an overweight woman (because as we all know, it's much more acceptable for a man to be a bit on the portly side than it is for a woman) or what it's like to experience pregnancy, there's a slim chance he's going to be able to empathize without you clueing him in to how you're feeling and what you're going through.

It can also be hard to give up control of some things in your life, but pregnancy is a time when you must be willing to ask for and accept help from your partner. Not only will it make things easier for you, but it will bring you closer together. The only way your partner can do any of the work involved with your pregnancy is to do things for you right now. He can't carry the baby around or take over your nausea. He can listen and encourage you. He can carry the laundry and lift the toddler into the high chair for you. He can rub your back and bring you strawberry smoothies when you want them. Let him do these things—it will make you both feel good.

Pregnancy is the beginning of your time together as parents. Allow your partner to be a part of this by trusting him. He may not always be as sensitive as you would like, but most of the time, he means well and he loves you and wants to be part of your pregnancy.

"I did feel self-conscious at first, but my husband was wonderful. I told him that I just didn't feel sexy. He told me that I was even more beautiful now, knowing that we had really joined together in making life, and he loved me and I would always be sexy and beautiful to him. My advice is to be honest. If you just turn away from your partner, he might not understand and feel rejected and think it's his fault. Have faith that he loves you. Tell him how you feel. Probably, his opinion of you hasn't changed a bit, and if it has, it's for the better."—Vanessa R.

"It's hard for me to get undressed around my husband when I'm pregnant. But he thinks I'm beautiful no matter what size I am. I just tell him to be patient with me. I have to get used to my growing body so I can feel comfortable around him."—Dana W.

"I still feel like my husband looks at me and goes 'Ugh!' He tells me otherwise, that it is just part of being a mommy, but I want to feel and look sexy for him. I don't know what my husband sees when he looks at me, although he hugs me and says that he sees a beautiful woman carrying his child. I decided that I have to trust that, whether he means it in his soul or not. I firmly believe that communication on every level begins with trust. I think women have a hard time trusting their vanity, their emotions to their husbands, because we don't think that they could possibly understand exactly how we feel."—Cheryl H.

"If you are intimate enough with this person to have sex with him, you shouldn't feel funny about talking with [him]!"—DeAnn R.

"During my first pregnancy, I was very self-conscious about the extra weight I was carrying and worried what my husband would think. When I finally got the courage to discuss it with him, he was surprised I felt so bad. I wish I had shared my concerns sooner."—Beth U.

"One of the things that has helped me the most is to have a loving and supportive partner. My husband loves my curves and tells me so often, even as he supports me in my [postpartum] efforts to lose weight for my health."—Carla R.

Your Friends and Family

Friends and family are great people to lean on. Your parents are going to be grandparents, so this is an exciting time for them, as well. Your parents love you just the way you are, and their support can help you get through difficult times. Your mom knows what it's like to be pregnant, and even if she is not the same size as you, she at least has been through it all and has some understanding of how you're feeling. If your close female relatives (mom, sister, aunt, grandmother, etc.) have body shapes similar to yours, they can reassure you about how you look and how you will get through the pregnancy. Reaching out to your family can be an important way to get the support you need. While husbands and friends are wonderful, there's nothing like knowing you have the support of a community of women inside your family.

Girlfriends are terrific people to take with you when shopping for maternity clothes, especially those girlfriends who have had babies. They can help you decide what fits, what's attractive, and just how much you need to buy. Some women are uncomfortable talking to their thinner friends about their plus-size pregnancy issues. Sure, your girlfriend knows what it's like to have swollen ankles and cravings, but she might not know what it's like to worry about whether the ultrasound tech is going to be able to get a clear shot of the baby through a bigger stomach. How you deal with this depends on your friendship. Some girlfriends are there for you no matter what you go through, and size is no object. These are the friends you can tell anything to and who will support you through thick and thin (so to speak). Rely on these friends to get you through the tough times. Spill it to them, and know that you can't say anything that will make them love you less.

If you have other friends who simply don't understand what you're going through and don't have the sensitivity to help you deal with it, don't talk to them about your plus-size issues. You can still talk about your pregnancy and your joys and worries and ups and downs with them, but if you aren't comfortable sharing it all, you don't have to. Dr. McVey-Noble says, "If you have unsupportive family or friends, don't talk to them. It really is that simple. This is the time to nix negativity and to focus on the miracle occurring in your life. Stick with the positive people in your life and be positive."

"My friends and family are fantastic—no one has said a word about my weight because I don't have an issue with it."—Liz O.

"I have one friend who is the skinniest thing going. She has trouble keeping on weight. But I love her like a sister and had no qualms about telling her everything I was going through.

Size doesn't matter to us, and she supported me through everything, even if she didn't have personal experience with some of what I was going through."—Lee T.

"I got support from my family and friends. My sister had a baby six months before I did, and she was a great source of advice and comfort. My mother made me feel special by taking me shopping for maternity clothes and empathizing at the small selection that there is out there. Mom is larger, too, and she could really sympathize when I would see cute maternity outfits that just didn't come in my size."—Carla R.

"My mother is a heavy woman, and she was very understanding and helpful when I needed assistance."—Amelia M.

Your Health-Care Provider

If you have a good, comfortable relationship with your health-care provider or with nurses in the office, they can be excellent sources to turn to. Your health-care provider can help you understand that the changes and feelings you're experiencing are normal, which can be a helpful thing to hear when you're certain you've become a raving lunatic with a belly the size of a hot-air balloon. Going to your OB appointments and being honest about how you're feeling both physically and emotionally will let your provider know just what you've been experiencing. She is the expert on pregnancy, and there is nothing she hasn't heard before. You might be surprised at some of the solutions or suggestions that will help you feel better about yourself or feel comfortable physically.

You may find that you develop a good relationship with the aides or front-desk staff at your doctor's office, as well. While they are not medical experts, they do see an awful lot of pregnant women every day, and their friendly words of advice or support can really make you feel good when you need it.

"I always left my OB appointments feeling so good. The staff was so nice, and my doctor was the most-wonderful woman. She was larger and had two kids of her own, so I felt like I could really talk to her about anything I was going through. I've gone through a lot in that office—breaking down and crying when I was having secondary infertility, being elated about new pregnancies, terrified about C-sections, and upset about a miscarriage. Through it all, she has supported me, given me information, but also given me hugs."—Gail D.

Finding Online Support

There are a lot of options available for women who want to join online support groups. One popular type is a due-date club. The group is labeled with a month and year, and the women who join are all due in that month. This way, you're talking with women who are going through many of the same changes you are at about the same time. Some of these groups have longevity, with moms remaining friends long after birth as they share support about the different stages their children go through. To find a due-date club go to:

www.fertilethoughts.com

www.mothering.com

www.babyzone.com

www.justmommies.com

www.parentsplace.com

Another option is online support groups specifically for plus-size pregnant women. You can find groups at:

- *www.yourplussizepregnancy.com*, the companion site to this book.
- *www.babycenter.com*. (Go to the Community section. Click on "pregnancy under Bulletin Boards, and go from there or type *http//bbs.baby center.com/board/pregnancy/8404* into your browser's address bar.)
- *www.parentsplace.com* (direct link at the time of publication was

www.parentsplace.com/messageboards)

- *www.fertilityplus.org*. (Click on table of contents, and scroll to Fertility Resource Lists, direct link at the time of publication was *www.fertilityplus.org/bbw/*)
- You can also find groups at *www.yahoogroups.com* if you search for "BBW pregnancy," "plus-size pregnancy," or "overweight pregnancy."
- If you have Polycystic Ovarian Syndrome, there are a variety of PCOS support groups, including *www.soulcysters.net* and *www.pcossupport.org*.

If you've never belonged to an online group and are unfamiliar with how they work, these tips will help you:

- Read the group's rules so you understand what is permitted. (For example, some lists ask that you stick just to pregnancy or weight discussions, while others allow general chitchat.)
- Post to introduce yourself once you join.
- Read previous posts to the list so you can get a feel for what the group is like.
- Try to stay out of any heated discussions.
- Decide if you want to receive each e-mail individually, subscribe to a daily digest, or just read posts online.
- Join in gradually. You may be tempted to spill everything all at once, but it's usually a good idea to first find out if this is a place where you will feel comfortable and accepted before sharing deeply personal thoughts.
- Don't feel pressured into posting. There are lots and lots of people who join chat rooms or discussion boards and never make a peep. It's OK to just lurk and read what other people are saying.

Boards and listservs can be a great way to make contact with women you wouldn't be able to find or meet otherwise. It can be a little odd at first to read personal messages from strangers or to try to write something yourself without knowing any of the women there. But in general, lists like these are very friendly and welcoming. And particularly with pregnancy boards, people are always coming or going as they have babies or get pregnant, so you aren't the only new person to the list. What's nice about lists is that you can read the posts whenever it's convenient for you, and you can either become an active member, posting regularly yourself, or just lurk, reading the messages that are there and learning that there are people just like you going through similar things.

"I am a LiveJournal.com user. There are many communities regarding pregnancy. Most people on those communities are extremely supportive and have good tips and advice."—Becky A.

"I have found a great resource in Baby Center's iVillage message board for pregnant and overweight moms. With the support of the women on the iVillage message board, it has been a lot easier to realize that it's more likely that my pregnancy will be mostly uneventful than not."—Jill G.

"iVillage has some great boards for pregnancy. I was, and still am, on the Pregnant & Overweight/Overweight Moms board. The ladies on there are so wonderful and helped me so much during my pregnancy—and still do now that my daughter is here. They also have expecting clubs for the month you're expecting in."—Jennifer W.

"I did join OPSS-overweight pregnant support system online message board. It's nice to commiserate and share exciting times."—Jen R.

"I am part of a wonderful online support group called OPSS-L Overweight & Pregnant Support. It can be found at Yahoo Groups. I used to be consumed with worry day and night. These wonderful ladies who are going through virtually the same thing I am helped me realize that worry will not change the outcome of this pregnancy."—Richelle H.

"OPSS-L (*http://health.groups.yahoo.com/group/OPSS-L*). It seemed every time I had a burning question, someone would have asked it within the past few days."—Jeanie T.

"I belong to OPSS-L, and I actually have my own forum—currently 250 members—that deals with pregnancy, infertility, parenting, and related issues: *www.theob.net/board/*."—Liz O.

"I joined a 'Due in July' list. There are women of all shapes, sizes, nationalities, etc. We are still very close. It's comforting to talk to a group of women who are at the same stage in their pregnancies, and after the births, you'll have a group of women who all have babies the same age to compare weights, milestones, first teeth, first words, etc."—Andrea H.

"There is a group called OMOM and a related pregnancy group as well as an infertility group. I participated in the pregnancy group through most of my pregnancies and am currently in the OMOM group. A nice group of ladies where you can ask questions like 'Are you sure they will have gowns big enough for me?' and not be embarrassed."—Margie P.

12

Celebrating and Honoring Your Pregnancy

*Y*our pregnancy is a very special time. This is the beginning of your child's life and the beginning of your life as a mother. It's a time of anticipation, excitement, and nervousness. Not everyone can have a baby, and not all pregnancies are successful (due to miscarriage), so your pregnancy is truly a miracle.

Taking the time and making the effort to enjoy your pregnancy and focus on it will not only make you feel good about yourself now, but it will also help you preserve memories of it so that years from now you'll be able to look back on it with good feelings. Many plus-size women feel embarrassed about their pregnant bodies, but taking the time to savor your new shape and appreciate it can actually help you feel better about yourself and your situation.

Your pregnancy will last for only a short time. Try to enjoy it while you can. It's the only time in your child's life when you are completely connected—honor and cherish it.

Focus on Your Pregnancy

When you first find out you're pregnant, it's big news for you and your partner and immediate family. But you've got months of waiting to get through. The fact that you're going to have a baby starts to dim a little, and, if you're dealing with nausea, it can take a backseat to the discomfort you're experiencing. You're not about to forget you're pregnant, but it's easy to lose sight of the big picture.

Keeping your eye on the prize will not only help you weather the difficult moments of your pregnancy, but it will remind you to enjoy every second of it. Although pregnancy can seem trying when you're going through it, many women look back on it wistfully once it's over. So instead of getting bogged down in feeling sick, tired, fat, and sore, remember that every symptom you feel is part of the incredible miracle of your pregnancy.

To help yourself focus on the joys of your pregnancy, try these tips:

Track your progress
Buy a book, such as *A Child Is Born* by Lennart Nilsson, or computer program (see Appendix) that shows you your baby's development each week. You'll get to see the growth of arms and legs and changes in size. Seeing what your baby really looks like each week can help make it all seem much more real. And opening the book or using the program can give you a real sense of connection to a baby that you may not be able to feel yet.

Exercise
Choose a form of exercise that allows you to focus on your body and enjoy it. Yoga is an excellent choice during pregnancy, and the mental component will help you concentrate on your body and the amazing changes you are experiencing. (See Chapter 6 for more information on choosing exercise.)

Relax
Make time to take a bath, get a foot massage, have your nails done, or

simply lay down and feel your baby kicking. Get in tune with your body and what it's doing, and you'll feel more connected to the baby. A lot of women see pregnancy as a time to get everything done that they think they won't have time for once the baby comes, but the truth is that you can overdo it. This is a time when your body needs rest.

Get in contact with your body

Touch your changing stomach, and get to know its shape and curves. Rubbing your stomach can calm you and make you feel more in touch with the baby and your pregnancy. You might feel awkward about looking at yourself in the mirror, but if you focus on your growing belly, you can enjoy the changes you see happening. Sometimes just sitting quietly and just *being* can be a useful way to get in tune with your body.

Listen to your pregnancy

You can purchase or rent a Doppler for use at home, so you can listen to your baby's heartbeat any time. Hearing the heartbeat can be reassuring and soothing.

"I had a book that showed in detail how my baby looked and what was happening at each stage of the pregnancy. I would also write in a journal about changes that were taking place with me, either physically or emotionally. You tend to forget the details of what it was like to be pregnant. This helps to remind you later."—Beth U.

"Sometimes my husband and I would just lie in bed and watch the baby's movements."—Lee T.

"I would lie in bed and just feel my baby move inside me. I loved that, and it was really cool when the baby got big enough to where I could see my belly move when he did. I would sit in bed and laugh for an hour. That always got me in a good mood."—Shannan E.

"We rented a fetal Doppler from *www.babybeat.com*, and every night before bed, we would listen to the heartbeat with our three-and-a-half-year-old. That was a wonderful way to enjoy the pregnancy and share it with her."—Andrea H.

Celebrate and Remember Your Pregnancy

Some women find themselves avoiding cameras and trying to leave virtually no trace of their pregnancies. Others feel so miserable during their pregnancies that they say they want absolutely nothing to remind them of this difficult time. Your pregnancy is important not only to you and your spouse, but to your baby. Keeping some tangible memories of it will help show your child what a special time it was to you and will help you remember the good feelings you had while pregnant.

Keep a pregnancy journal

Buy a pregnancy journal or use a blank book or open a computer file or start a blog. Record your thoughts and feelings, as well as changes in your body. Milestone events to record include telling your partner about your pregnancy, sharing the news with other people, first hearing the heartbeat, outgrowing your clothes, the first kick, choosing a name, ultrasounds, and the beginning of labor. A journal is also a good place to work through the ups and downs you're dealing with. Writing about how you feel can help you understand and resolve conflicting emotions. Some women find that writing in a journal helps them understand exactly what is bothering them and find ways to cope with it.

"I have started a pregnancy journal. If I remember to write in it, I think it will be neat to look back in. I do avoid writing in the weight and measurements section, though."—Jill G.

"I have been working on a book for the baby called *My Pregnancy*. You can order it on amazon.com. It is a record book of your symptoms, feelings, ultrasounds, showers, and other memorable pregnancy moments."—Jennifer N.

"The best thing I did was to keep a journal of how I felt while pregnant and the changes I went through. You think you'll never forget, but you do. Having a written record of it helps me to remember what it was like, and it's something I can share with my kids one day."
—Beth U.

Take photos

Even if you're a person who tries to avoid cameras on your best days, you should make sure there are at least some photos of your pregnancy. For one thing, you'll forever feel better about your postpregnancy body when you compare it to your pregnant self. And your child will want to see what he or she looked like as part of you. If you don't take any pictures, you will send your child the message that you were ashamed of how you looked or thought your pregnancy wasn't important.

"I love the photos of daddy and mommy's hands on the belly! Every photo I have during those nine months has someone 'holding' the baby, listening to the baby, or kissing the baby."—Vanessa R.

"I would love to get professional pregnancy pictures done, but we'll have to see if my belly ever actually looks pregnant."—Jennifer N.

"Every time I had a doctor's appointment, my husband would take a profile picture of me in front of the office. It made for a neat retrospective of my changing belly after we were all done. I had pictures taken about three weeks before I delivered. I was wearing a soft white nightgown, and in a lot of the profile shots, you can see through the gown and see my belly. I love those pictures, and I felt so incredibly beautiful taking them."—Carla R.

"Take pictures. Make sure that someone takes lots of pictures of you and your growing belly. You may feel weird about it, but later you will treasure seeing your pregnancy glow and your overly rounded belly."—Ali S.

"With my second pregnancy, we took family pregnancy pictures with my husband and four-year-old daughter with a professional photographer. We did nude (from the waist up) pictures with me and my husband, pictures with my daughter and my belly, pictures of my daughter painting my naked belly, pictures of the three of us and the belly, etc. It was wonderful and great for my self-esteem."—Andrea H.

"My sister-in-law is a photographer and tried to talk me into doing them in each pregnancy. At thirty weeks in my last pregnancy, I decided I should document my belly, even if it wasn't a picture-perfect one. I did pictures. I made her use a digital camera so there wouldn't be any developers giggling about them, but they turned out gorgeous. I still like to pull them out and look at them. My belly isn't perfect—it droops on the bottom and has an appendecto-my scar over my bellybutton, but it was a safe harbor for my four sweet babies, and I am glad to have pictures. I liked the pictures so much that at thirty-seven weeks, I had more taken with my three children. I have one framed on my dresser with the three kids touching my bare belly. I resisted touching up even the scar on my belly. It's who I am, and I like it!"—Margie P.

Wear outward signs of pregnancy

Wearing maternity clothes (see Chapter 9) can help you feel and look pregnant. Some women like to wear shirts that make it clear they are pregnant. There are other ways to show the world, too. Consider buying pregnancy jewelry from *www.twinklelittlestar.com/us/pregnancy-jewelry.html*. You can also find a variety at *www.attachmentscatalog.com/gifts/jsilver.html*, including the Pregnancy Angel pin and earrings and pendants with babies on them. See the Appendix for even more pregnancy jewelry choices.

Preserve ultrasounds

Ask your doctor or midwife to make a DVD or video for you of your baby's ultrasound and for printouts of screen shots. Many women keep these as their baby's first pictures and begin an album with them.

Celebrate milestones

There are many big days in your pregnancy. Don't let them pass by. For example, celebrate the first kick with a shopping trip to buy things for the nursery. Or go out to dinner after your first ultrasound. Have a day out with girlfriends to celebrate your first shopping trip for maternity clothes. Some women perform religious observances throughout their pregnancies, such as lighting candles or saying special prayers.

"My husband and I always had lunch together after every doctor's appointment during my first pregnancy. It was a nice way to spend some time together and think about the baby."—Lee T.

"Every woman who becomes pregnant should give thanks to whatever God they worship because pregnancy is the one true miracle in human life."—Sharon L.

Mark each month

Make note of when you pass from one month of pregnancy to the next. Do something special for each. This can be as small as writing in big letters on your calendar what month you've moved to or taking a photo each time. The months will go by more quickly than you expect, and if you do something special to remember each month of your pregnancy, it will stop it all from just slipping past you.

Get a belly cast made

Some women are horrified at the thought of someone making a cast of their pregnant belly, but others want to preserve their shape. If it's something you would feel comfortable doing, you can order a kit online (*www.proudbody.com* or *www.castingmiracles.com*) and do it at home, or you may be able to find a local artist who can cast it for you.

> "With my first pregnancy, I did a belly cast. That was a lot of fun."—Andrea H.
>
> "I think belly casts are a cool idea, but I would have been way too self-conscious because of my size."—Julie M.

Make substitutions

So you can't drink alcohol, are limiting your caffeine intake, and can't get into a hot tub. Instead of feeling deprived, make substitutions that you will enjoy. Buy an assortment of decaffeinated teas, drink sparkling cider, take long hot showers, buy chocolate milk, or make something silly like Kool-Aid®. There are plenty of ways to treat yourself without breaking the restrictions your doctor or midwife has given you.

Get Your Partner Involved in Your Pregnancy

It can be difficult for your partner to feel as involved in your pregnancy since he can't experience it in the same up-close and personal way you do. Getting him involved and interested can make you feel good about yourself and the pregnancy and help him connect with the baby and the changes happening to your body. It's also an important way for you to connect with each other. Pregnancy might be something that is happening only to your body, but it is something that is happening in your relationship and is going to have long-lasting effects for both of you. Consider these ways to get him involved:

Ask for massages

Ask him to rub your feet, your shoulders, your back and your belly—whatever is sore, achy, or tired. Putting his hands on your body will help him connect to the changes you are going through and appreciate the beauty pregnancy creates. If you feel self-conscious about just whipping out your big pregnant belly, have him rub it through a thin shirt or nightgown. You'll still get the benefits of connecting without feeling completely exposed.

Talk to him

Tell him how you're feeling, what you're experiencing, and what you're thinking. He can't know if you don't tell him. When you describe what you're feeling physically and emotionally, it will not only help him understand, it will make you feel closer to him because you've shared private parts of yourself.

Work on plans together

Talk about arranging the nursery or picking out a crib. Discuss your plans for day care, ask his advice about what clothes look good on you, and have him come with you to buy a baby monitor. (You can be sure he'll get excited about technology!) Get him involved and delegate some jobs to him. When he makes decisions that impact the baby, he will feel like an important part of the pregnancy. And when you discuss things and plan them together, you solidify your bond with each other and lay the groundwork for future teamwork together as parents.

> "When my husband was working on wallpapering the nursery for our first child, I remember it gave me this really nice warm feeling, like he was taking active steps to prepare for the baby, and in some way, like he was taking care of me, too."—Lee T.

Go to classes

Encourage him to go with you to prenatal education classes. Having him there is important so that he can learn how to help you through labor and what to expect. It's also important because it solidifies your image together as a team. You're going to get through labor and delivery together, and the classes will help you think that way about it. There are many other classes available beyond birth preparation, such as infant CPR, breastfeeding, baby care, and early pregnancy classes. Attending these together can also help you feel connected and prepared.

> "With my first pregnancy, we went to a six-week childbirth class and went out to dinner alone before each class. It just made it feel more special, and I fondly remember those nights now that we never go out."—Brenda Z.

Make time for each other

With the birth of the baby just around the corner, pregnancy is a good time to plan some time alone together. Once the baby comes, you'll be busy, and even after things settle down, it will be hard to leave the baby. Plan some special nights out, or take a short trip together. Being alone together will give you time to talk and connect and feel close to one another.

13

It's Showtime:
Labor and Delivery

*G*iving birth to your baby is the moment you've been waiting for. It's what your whole pregnancy has been leading up to. In this chapter, we will again be using the medical definitions for the words overweight and obese, as they were defined in Chapter 7.

Childbirth is meant to be a time of joy, not a time of embarrassment, worry, or fear. Most plus-size women have normal childbirth or normal C-sections (discussed in Chapter 14) without any problems. Some women do encounter difficulties, and understanding what those are in advance can help you be knowledgeable and prepared if necessary.

Finding Childbirth Classes

Childbirth classes are an important part of your pregnancy. If this is your first pregnancy, you probably have a lot of questions and uncertainties about labor and delivery, as well as postpartum recovery. Childbirth classes will give you the information you crave. Finding a class that is right can take some work. There are some basic types of classes to consider:

Lamaze

The Lamaze method teaches breathing and relaxation techniques and encourages you to rely on a labor partner for support, relaxation assistance, and massage. The goal is natural childbirth, but the methods can be helpful no matter how you give birth.

Bradley

This method stresses the importance of prenatal fitness and nutrition. It relies on deep breathing and looking inward during labor.

Hypnobirthing

These classes use hypnosis to program deep relaxation into your mind for use during labor.

Combination

Combination classes teach a variety of methods and possibilities so that the woman can decide which technique she is most comfortable with, or use different techniques as needed throughout her labor.

VBAC

Vaginal Birth after Caesarean classes are designed to help women who have had a previous C-section prepare for a vaginal birth. They focus on strategies for moving labor along and pain and relaxation techniques.

Childbirth Refresher

Women who have already given birth once before know the basics, but might want some reminders about specific techniques or strategies.

While it doesn't matter which type of childbirth class you attend, what matters is that you *do* go. Many of the women interviewed for this book did not go to any type of childbirth preparation class with their first child or subsequent children. Childbirth class can not only help you manage the pain and be more informed, it can reduce your risk of C-section by teaching you how to work with your body. It's important to talk to your health-care provider about his or her preferences regarding the choices presented to you in class (such as internal and external monitoring) and to take a tour of the hospital or birth center where you will give birth so you know what to expect there.

Jane Hanrahan, president-elect of the International Childbirth Education Association (ICEA, *www.icea.org*) believes childbirth classes are essential for plus-size women because of the statistical likelihood of longer labors and C-sections (see later in this chapter for information). She says, "In my opinion, the reason for longer labors and C-sections in larger women is that they can't get into that upright position and let gravity do its work." Taking a childbirth preparation class can help you learn how to maximize gravity, deal with pain, and help your body work to get the baby born.

Hanrahan says it is essential that plus-size women be introduced to a variety of positions and methods so they can try any or all of them if needed. She recommends an ICEA-approved combination childbirth class that teaches a variety of methods. "Do not choose a class that is focused only on natural childbirth. Some Bradley and Lamaze classes don't even mention pain relief. You then have no idea what your options are. Go into childbirth with an open mind, knowing your alternatives. Know the risks and benefits of your options so that if you need to make a choice, you are prepared. If you have information, you are more likely to help yourself."

Many women do enjoy childbirth classes because it gives them an opportunity to spend time with their partner focusing on the birth and also offers an opportunity to get to know other women who are expecting their babies around the same time.

However, childbirth classes can also feel like a time when you see how you measure up. You might find yourself sitting in class and comparing yourself to the other women and wondering, "Are her thighs bigger than mine? Does she look pregnant while I just look fat?" Hanrahan says, "It is really important to understand that most women have body-image issues during pregnancy no matter what their size. You're not alone." In childbirth classes, the other women are not as deeply critical of your body as you are. Every woman in the room (except the instructor) is pregnant, and it's pretty certain that every woman there is feeling a bit ungainly. The instructor is not there to critique you or anyone else. She's there to give you information and help you with questions or concerns. If you have questions that you want to ask, but are embarrassed about, go up to her at the end of class and speak with her privately.

Hanrahan says that she has never met or observed a childbirth instructor who was not size-friendly (although she knows this doesn't mean they don't exist), but suggests you call ahead and ask if it's a real concern. In addition to general size-friendliness, she says if you have concerns about seating and comfort during the class, say so. "When you call to schedule the class, find out where it is located and what kind of setting it is. Some classrooms have only pillows on the floor. Others have folding chairs. I use couches and seat three people to a couch. We're used to accommodating a variety of needs. Some women come to class on bed rest and have to lay down for the entire thing. Some women are in wheelchairs or casts. There's nothing we can't work with."

Depending on the type of class you take, you might find yourself on the floor with your partner and some pillows, practicing positions, breathing, and exercises. Don't feel self-conscious—everyone else in the room is trying to maneuver their big bellies onto the floor and into position, too. Some classes also give you the opportunity to try out a birth ball (and you should know that most are designed to hold up to 1,000 pounds so you're not going to break it). If you don't want to use the ball in front of other women, wait until the class is over to give it a try.

Hanrahan also points out that an important component of child-birth classes is nutrition. "I do a nutrition exercise where I have you write down everything you ate that day—women and men. We look at the diet to make sure you're getting enough protein, calcium, iron, and so on. It's not about seeing who ate cookies. If I had a woman who was uncomfortable with that exercise, I would teach that information in a different way. A less-experienced teacher might not know this, so find out how long an instructor has been teaching when you sign up."

The bottom line about childbirth classes, according to Hanrahan, is, "Everybody's welcome."

"I went to a labor and delivery class, and I was among mothers-to-be that ranged in size from bigger than me to way smaller, so I was comfortable. The instructor took the time to give us larger students methods out of the norm that would help us ease labor pains and aid in delivery that were aimed at us and our situation. It really helped and made me feel more comfortable, and it really helped during labor."—Vanessa R.

"The instructor was very considerate. When I was worried about popping the birth ball, she assured me I would have to weigh a lot more than I did to do any damage to it. She also showed me some ways to use a chair or the bed instead."—Carla R.

"We went to a combination childbirth class, and I was definitely the largest woman there, but I didn't feel uncomfortable. Most pregnant women I have found are thinking mostly about themselves and their baby, not about what someone else in the class looks like. It's a bonding experience for you and your spouse, too."—Jen R.

"I went to a combination class and was in a room with thin pregnant women. I felt uncomfortable and kept comparing myself to them. But I'm glad I went because I did learn a lot."—Lee T.

"I took a childbirth prep class. I was the biggest there. I did feel a little self-conscious, but my husband was with me, and it was better with him there."—Deb P.

"I was the only heavy person in the class, and there were a few things they wanted me to do on the floor that were not easy, so I did the best I could."—Jennifer H.

Being Honest About Your Weight

When you go to the hospital or work with a midwife, it's important to be honest with the staff about your weight. Certain medications may not work well if you don't give an accurate number. You may be asked your weight at several points. When you're first admitted, they'll ask for your weight and if you need or want anesthesia of any kind. The anesthesiologist may ask you again later. Some women have no problem providing this number in front of their spouse or partner, but if you feel uncomfortable, ask him to step out of the room while you share this information.

If you want to prevent every last resident and anesthesiologist who walk in the door from asking you how much you weigh, let your labor nurse know you're a little uncomfortable talking about your weight. They don't need to ask you this—it's in your chart, and your nurse has your number. She can easily communicate this to anyone who needs to know it. Labor nurses completely understand that pregnant women (of all sizes!) may not want their weight broadcast over the PA system.

Birth Comfort Measures

Be sure to read other pregnancy books for information about comfort measures during labor such as massage, breathing, positioning, and counterpressure. All the regular methods are good ones to try and should not be affected by your size. Some women find that they can't completely rest their weight on their birth partner or labor coach (or worry that they shouldn't).

If you need help supporting your body weight during contractions, ask the staff for a walker. Walkers have rubber feet and will support your entire body weight if you need to lean on them during labor. One position that might work is squatting and using the walker to support yourself as you do so. Another option is to have your attendant kneel on the bed, and then you lean on him or her. This will provide a completely stable situation and will allow the bed to take some of your weight. You might also put the birth ball on the bed and lean forward over it.

Hanrahan points out that most hospitals have squatting bars that can be very useful and says, "Hospital beds have 100 different positions. There are a lot of ways to get into different positions using the things available to you. You may be more apt to have a C-section, but try all these other things first." (See Chapter 14 for more information about C-sections.)

If your labor coach, doula, or birth attendant is having trouble holding you up as you push, ask him or her to sit behind you on the bed. This will provide much more even support and will be easier on both your bodies than trying to stand next to you and hold your back up with one hand. You can also raise the hospital bed and put pillows behind you.

Birth doula Andrea Henderson says, "Some women are worried about putting their weight on the birth ball or getting on their hands and knees for fear of how they look in that position to the hospital staff or their husbands or others who might see them. Also, some of them are too self-conscious to get in the tub, naked from the waist down. It is important for plus-size women to know that the doctors and nurses have seen it all. I would encourage women to work on feeling positive about their bodies before their birth experience so they are comfortable enough to try different positions and the many labor-coping techniques."

Hanrahan says that plus-size women worry about using the birth ball. "They worry they will be too heavy. Also, it's important to understand that when you are pregnant, your center of gravity is off, so even women who weigh 100 pounds are intimidated by the birth ball. It won't pop under your weight, and when you are on the ball you are never left alone. Someone is always there to support you, so don't worry."

Hygiene

When you're in labor or right after you give birth, you might feel plain icky. You're sweating, you've got all kinds of bodily fluids going in every direction, and you're uncomfortable. Some plus-size women feel extremely uncomfortable about being sweaty or dirty while in labor or afterward. The first thing to remember is none of this has anything to do with your size. Labor and delivery are hard work, and every woman is going to experience similar situations and feelings.

Your partner can bring you some water and wipe you with a wet cloth (this can feel quite soothing) where you are sweaty. Your labor nurse is there to assist you, and she can help you clean up anything anywhere on your body. (She's seen it all, so don't worry.) You can also take a shower during labor, and your labor nurse or partner can help you with that.

Dealing with Hospital Staff

The hospital staff is completely accustomed to seeing and working with all kinds of bodies. They have truly seen it all, so you don't need to worry that they will be shocked or horrified by you. They are there to care for you and help you through this. They should treat you with respect and dignity, and in most cases, you will find this to be the type of treatment you receive. If you aren't treated well, you have every right to speak up, request that someone else care for you, or complain. Every hospital has a patient advocate department, staff members who are assigned to make sure patients are treated well and to handle complaints. You can ask to see a patient advocate at any time during your stay.

It is hoped that the care you receive will be kind and compassionate. If it's not, it's important to at least understand some of the underlying reasons. Some medical personnel have been trained to be concerned about overweight patients who are in labor. They are on the lookout for problems or complications. You do want your care providers to look out for potential problems—that's why they're there. But sometimes we have observed that medical personnel (especially those that are less experienced) have anxiety responses to this extra responsibility. They're worried about making sure everything goes well for you and end up acting gruff or hostile in reaction to the stress, not as a reaction to your size. This same thing can happen when treating patients with other conditions that might be of potential concern, so it's not always a size-acceptance issue. Some patients who have had this problem with their health-care providers find that after delivery, when everything has gone smoothly, the health-care providers no longer act the same way and are much friendlier. This is just something to keep in mind (but is by no means an excuse) should you feel as though you aren't being treated as kindly as you would like.

It's also important to understand that your labor nurse is your absolute best friend while you are in the labor wing, and many are very, very protective of "their" moms. Your nurse is there to make sure you are physically *and* emotionally comfortable. If someone treats you poorly and she hears it, there's a good chance she will say something (possibly out of your earshot). She has seen women of all sizes give birth and has no doubts about your abilities. She is there to get you through it all, so rely on her if you can.

The hospital staff is used to seeing naked bodies and won't give any thought to seeing yours. If you're uncomfortable with the amount of exposure, ask for a sheet or additional gown to cover yourself. You'll probably find, however, once you're in labor, you will reach a point where personal modesty becomes unimportant because you're working so hard to get the baby out.

After the birth, you may also feel uncomfortable trying to nurse with people coming in and out of your room. Feel free to ask to have the curtain drawn or the door shut if you want some privacy. If you are seeing your baby down at the nursery, they may have screens they can move or curtains they can pull to offer you some privacy.

One thing many women interviewed for this book mentioned was the number of people it took to lift them if they had to be moved from a gurney to an operating-room table. What you must understand is that it *always* takes several people to move any patient, and you aren't an exception. The hospital most likely has a set policy regarding the minimum number of staff required to lift any patient, both for the patient's and the staff's safety. If you suddenly see four or five people about to lift you, don't feel shocked or embarrassed.

"I caught (even in my drugged state) a look pass between my Ob/Gyn and a nurse when he told me to move over and acted like it was my size preventing me from scooting over onto an operating-room table. He seemed to forget that I was literally numb from my neck down and my arms were pinned down. I just kept telling myself that I would never see most of these people again."—Julie M.

"I was self-conscious about them lifting me from the surgery table to the other bed, but there wasn't much I could do but hope they could do it."—Peggy M.

"I remembered every mom, including supermodels, is self-conscious about her body during labor and delivery. So that got me over it."—Liz R.

"It took six medical staff to hoist me from the trolley onto the bed in the operating theater, something that worried me because I didn't want to be responsible for injuring any of them."—Sharon L.

"Remember, every pregnant woman goes through this, no matter what size. And no matter how skinny they are, they still look like hell while they're in labor. Everybody does."—Ali S.

"With my first pregnancy, my bed wheels broke so they couldn't roll me into the OR, then the rail broke, and they couldn't get the side down for me to get out of bed, but I couldn't feel my legs anyhow because of my meds. They had to have four people lift me onto the other bed—humiliating!"—Angie G.

"Getting from the surgery table to your bed, it was a piece of cake. It took ten seconds, and it was over. I was so worried about them having to lift me, but they do it so you don't have to be lifted. I even asked, and the nurse said that should not even be a worry for me, to just think about my baby coming. When you are having contractions or anything like that, you really and truly will not care what anyone sees. People told me this for years, and I never believed it until I was in the situation."—Jennifer H.

"With my second child, a nurse in triage asked if I could lie on the exam table—it is a steel table, for goodness sake! What did she think was going to happen?"—Margie P.

Hospital Equipment and Supplies

The biggest complaint by women interviewed for this book is about hospital gowns. They just don't fit. What you need to remember is that hospital gowns really fit no one! They're designed to create easy access should the staff need to get to your body; they're really not meant to provide complete coverage (as you will note from that nasty draft up the back). Other hospital equipment may not fit you well, either. Let's go through the list of potential problems and how to solve them:

Gowns

If they give you one that is too small or doesn't cover enough, ask for a bigger one. If they don't have any other size or if a bigger one doesn't help, ask for a second gown. Put the first one on open in the back, then put the second one on over it, open in the front. You will be completely covered. You can also bring your own nightgowns or long, loose, short-sleeve button-front shirts to use. If you have a vaginal birth, you can probably put your own clothes back on soon afterward. (Don't expect your prepregnancy clothes to fit just yet though.)

Blood-pressure cuffs

Just as at the doctor's office, you may need to request a larger cuff. Hospitals will have these (unlike some doctor's offices where they may not), so all you need to do is ask. Blood-pressure machines are common-place now and do have optional larger cuffs, although they may not have one for each machine, meaning one will have to be located.

Fetal monitors

These monitors record the baby's heartbeat, as well as your contractions. If you have external fetal monitoring, there is the possibility that the belt may not fit you, although most of them are expandable. If this is the case, ask the nurse if the belt can be extended using a roll of gauze. Intermittent monitoring with a handheld Doppler is possible, but it doesn't give your doctor a complete ongoing record, and it could miss periods of problems with the heartbeat. Most labor wings track monitors with centralized computer stations, allowing the computer to evaluate and create a digital record of the baby's heart rate and activity. Intermittent external monitoring fails to provide these benefits. External monitors are highly sensitive and work for women of all sizes.

Internal monitors (attached to the baby's scalp) are used much less often because of the excellent quality of external monitors. They're only used when an external monitor, for whatever reason, is not providing continuous results or there is a serious risk to the baby. If the problem is that you're not getting consistent results, then you may be moving around too much. Reducing your activity can improve your readings. (There's a trade-off here, of course—moving around can help labor to progress.) Internal monitors mean your water must be broken, and once this happens, you have a time limit on when you must give birth or face a C-section.

Doctors will recommend monitoring for larger women because there is an increased risk of problems during labor (slowed labor—see later in this chapter—and the need for Pitocin). Monitoring may be a good idea, but some women just don't want it. Discuss this with your doctor. Just because you're larger doesn't necessarily mean that your baby must be constantly monitored. If you're induced or using pain medication or anesthesia, a monitor will be required in most cases.

In the past, internal and external monitoring have been reported to lead to increased C-section rates (because they restrict movement), but recent research shows this is not the case. The trouble with many of the studies that showed an increased C-section rate was that the problem is often "physician distress" rather than the baby being in distress. Misinterpretation of the monitor information by inexperienced physicians and nurses, and a failure to use conservative measures to get things on track prior to using C-section, forceps, or vacuum extraction, causes many C-sections. Simple measures such as placing the mother on her side, increasing the IV drip rate, giving a small dose of oxygen to the mother, correcting low blood pressure induced by an epidural, or decreasing the Pitocin drip rate, may be all that's necessary. Sometimes fetal sleep cycles or pain medication may wrongly give the impression that the baby is in trouble, again leading to overreaction by the doctor or nurse.

Sometimes, when fetal monitoring results are of concern, but are not dangerous, your doctor may use an acoustic stimulator. This is a small device that sends sound at specific decibels through your abdomen, which stimulates parts of the baby's brain. If the oxygen level in the baby's brain is normal, this acoustical stimulation will show a response on the fetal monitoring and will be reassuring. You may feel the baby suddenly move when the stimulator is turned on. This movement is also reassuring. The acoustic stimulator does not harm or injure the baby, and its use has reduced the need for C-sections when the fetal monitor pattern is of concern.

There are other technologies used to monitor babies in labor. Fetal-scalp sampling is a technique during which a small drop of the baby's blood is obtained from his or her scalp and analyzed to detect a low oxygen level, though this is rarely used today. Another technique, called pulse oximetry, involves placing an electrode through the birth canal next to the baby's skin and measuring the oxygen saturation (the percent of the blood that is "saturated" with oxygen). It's not widely used, and its place in fetal monitoring is not well established.

In addition to the external fetal monitor, another external sensor is placed on the mother's abdomen to record the uterine contractions. It senses the change in the contour or shape of the mother's abdomen when the uterus contracts. In addition to tracking the frequency and duration of the contractions, it allows doctors to see the baby's reactions to contractions (by comparing the results from the two monitors you can see how the baby reacts at the time of a contraction). In plus-size moms, the monitor used to measure contractions may not work as effectively. Also, the external monitoring device does not give any information about the strength or power of the contraction for any women. An intrauterine pressure catheter may be inserted if the external monitor is not getting accurate results. This is inserted through the vaginal canal and is placed next to the baby. It allows a very accurate measurement of the frequency, duration, and strength of the contractions. It may also be used to infuse fluid into the uterine cavity. This is called amnioinfusion.

Amnioinfusion is used when there is not enough amniotic fluid around the umbilical cord, and it becomes compressed during a uterine contraction. The infusion of fluid restores the "fluid" cushion around the cord. It is also used when the baby has had a bowel movement in utero (which is more common with older gestational-age babies, babies that are past their due date, and moms who have hypertension). Early bowel movements are made up of a thick green substance called meconium, and may cause a problem if the baby inhales it at the time of birth. The infusion of fluid dilutes the meconium, making it less dangerous should the baby inhale it at the time of delivery.

It's important to discuss the fetal monitoring issue with your health-care provider before you go into labor. It is also important to choose a health-care provider who is experienced in interpreting fetal monitors. Though not foolproof, one indication of a doctor's experience with this may be his C-section rate. C-section rates are very difficult to interpret. A rate might be high because the doctor mostly cares for high-risk pregnancies or because he or she practices in a rural area where the decision to do a C-section needs to be made as far in advance as possible. You should consider the primary rate—the number of first pregnancies that end in C-section. The national rate for this is 10 to 15 percent. A high C-section rate for a doctor with a regular OB practice in a modern hospital may be an indication that he or she is not skilled in reading and managing monitors and is thus performing unnecessary C-sections. An experienced OB can manage this technology without ruining, or greatly interfering with, your birth process. You both have the same goal—a healthy baby. Continuous monitoring can assure you and your doctor that everything is going well as you give birth vaginally.

IVs
Weight usually has no impact on the ability to get an IV inserted, and you don't need a special needle or equipment. If you know, however, that you've had difficulty in the past or if they try and fail to get it in, ask that they get an expert or someone experienced working with patients who have difficult-to-find veins.

Needle length
If you have epidural or spinal anesthesia, you probably don't need to worry about the needle not being long enough—this is an extremely rare occurrence. If you're concerned, ask the anesthesiologist to make sure there will be no problem.

Underwear and pads

After your birth, you may be given hospital-issue underwear that is made of stretchy mesh and some pads to wear to help deal with postpartum vaginal bleeding. If the underwear doesn't fit or is uncomfortable, throw it out and wear a pair of your own. You may want to bring your pads from home—hospital issue usually doesn't have adhesive or wings. Always brand makes pads specifically for sizes 14 and up, and you might find them to be perfect for the postpartum recovery period when you have a heavy flow.

Abdominal support garment

If you have a C-section (or sometimes with a vaginal birth), the staff may have you wear an abdominal support garment afterward. It looks like a giant leg brace and is meant to give your abdomen support so that you don't feel like your stomach is falling out. If they try to squeeze you into one that doesn't fit, ask them to take it off and get a larger one. You're not going to be comfortable if you're squeezed into it like a corset—and if you have a C-section, a too-tight support garment can actually push your hanging belly down over your incision causing a greater chance of infection or complications. If they don't have one that fits you, a nurse may be able to wrap a towel or sheet around you and secure it with safety pins (although some kind of stretchy material will work best, so it can be stretched around you, and the elastic will help to hold in your tummy), or you can hold a pillow in front of your tummy whenever you move.

Table size

Some women worry that if they need a C-section, they won't fit on the operating-room table. Not to worry—the staff is experienced in working with people of all sizes and the table will be big enough for you. You won't fall off or hang over the edge.

"The hospital undies they gave me to wear after the baby were way too small. I just used my own."—Shannan E.

"I did have some problems with the small cuffs at the hospital. Finally, one of the nurses said she could just take my pressure on the lower part of my arm since she was using the machine. Once I found that was possible, I just told the other nurses to take my pressure that way instead of the half-hour-long hunt for the bigger cuff."—Tammy M.

"To get a gown that covers, simply put one gown on the regular way, and put another gown on like a jacket. That way both sides are covered."—Ali S.

"The hospital gowns just didn't fit well. As soon as I delivered and was taken to my room, I changed into my own nursing gown that I brought from home. I also had a hard time fitting into the elastic mesh panties that they put the pads in after you give birth. I solved that problem by putting the pads in some of my old maternity underwear. I didn't care if they got stained since I threw them out anyway."—Carla R.

"Hospital gowns never fit. I was always pulling and tugging on them, trying to cover up the best I could."—Beth U.

"I was issued this hospital gown that was way too small. My behind hung out, and I felt horrible that nobody took the time to gauge my size and find an appropriate garment. I had to wear a blanket over my shoulders."—Richelle I I.

"When I was going to the OR for my C-section, I wore two gowns. Very embarrassing!"—Angie G.

"With my first baby, the nurse realized the tummy support thing wouldn't fit and wrapped a bath towel around me. With the second baby, they somehow stuffed me into it. It was uncomfortable, and the Velcro kept coming undone. Finally, I just took it off."—Lee T.

"For a C-section, the table is quite narrow, but they do everything possible so you will not fall off. That was a worry of mine laying there."—Jennifer H.

"The monitor that they put around your belly to monitor the baby's heart rate did not stay put because it just didn't fit right. I just had to be careful how I moved to keep it in contact in the right way. It was annoying."—Melissa S.

Vaginal Birth

Being plus-size doesn't mean you can't have a completely normal vaginal birth. And any doctor that tells you otherwise (unless you have other complications) is misinformed. There is no reason to schedule a planned C-section for an overweight first-time mom unless there are other conditions or problems involved. Some women have reported being worried about their endurance or physical ability to give birth. Birth is actually an involuntary process, and even a woman who is in a coma will give birth vaginally. This is something that your body knows how to do on its own. The more you can help it along, the better, but you don't need to be able to run a marathon to have a vaginal birth.

Squatting or knee-chest positions help to open the pelvis and might be effective for you. Use gravity to help you. Walk and move around during labor if possible. Try to avoid just laying in bed on your back throughout your labor.

A 2004 study from the University of North Carolina at Chapel Hill showed that overweight or obese women tend to have longer active labors (the time it takes to go from 4 cm dilation to 10). The study showed normal women took about 6.2 hours while overweight women took 7.5 hours on average, and obese women took an average of 7.9 hours. Overweight women tended to stall between 4 and 6 cm, while obese women stalled under 7 cm. A longer labor is not necessarily bad (except of course, for the endless pain and your desire to just get it over with!), but this study indicates that you and your doctor should take your weight into consideration before considering a C-section for failure to progress. Because your body naturally may have a longer labor, things might actually be progressing at a reasonable rate for you, whereas it might seem long when compared with smaller women. Be sure to talk to your doctor about this if you find that your labor falls into the situations described. If you can wait out the extra bit of time (which might not sound like a lot now, but can feel like a lifetime when you're going through it), your labor may get through the stalled period and then move along.

> "I was worried that delivery would be difficult because I was not in shape or strong enough. I just kept walking and being as active as I could, and it all worked out."—Vanessa R.
>
> "I thought the delivery might be extra hard. It was fine, but long."—Liz R.
>
> "I did worry that it would make labor harder. I personally found this to be a myth. Since I weighed more with the last two babies than with the first and each labor got easier, I don't think weight is a factor here."—Michelle C.
>
> "After my first birth, I was impressed with my body's ability to deliver a baby. I didn't worry about anything the rest of the pregnancies. As a nonathletic person, I was really impressed with my body in a way I had never been before."—Margie P.

Breech Birth

If your baby is in breech position in your last trimester (rear end pointing down), your health-care provider may tell you not to worry because this is quite common around weeks thirty-two to thirty-four of pregnancy. A baby that is breech at thirty-seven weeks, however, is likely to stay that way. A University of Montreal study showed that when obese women have breech presentation, they are more likely to require a C-section. Recent research shows that breech babies have fewer complications if they are delivered by scheduled C-section (before labor begins). Breech delivery is no longer commonly taught to medical students, but it is sometimes possible to turn a baby while still in the uterus. This is called external cephalic version (ECV) and is done at thirty-seven to thirty-eight weeks. Labor-inhibiting drugs are administered beforehand to prevent the mother from going into early labor in response to the technique. The health-care provider manipulates the baby from outside the abdomen and tries to turn it. ECV is usually less successful in plus-size women or when the baby is large, but you should discuss it with your health-care provider if your baby is breech.

Induction

Some women and doulas report doctors inducing labor in larger women simply because they believed their size meant the baby would be too large to go to term. "I've heard of women being induced because they might have a big baby because they are big women, only to have a six-pound peanut to take home," points out birth doula Andrea Henderson.

If your doctor suggests induction, ask some hard questions. Why is he or she recommending this? If it's because the doctor believes your baby is going to be large, what test results indicate that and how reliable are they? (Ultrasound predictions are not very accurate near the end of pregnancy, and fundal height may measure large in larger women even if the baby isn't that big.) If your doctor believes your baby is very large and that induction is the best route, you need to weigh your options and the evidence he or she has presented. Waiting to go into labor may mean having to delivery a very large baby—or it could mean going into labor tomorrow with a normal-size baby. There's no way to know for sure when you're going to have the baby and how big he or she will be. If you do wait and deliver a big baby, it is likely your delivery will be more difficult and problems such as shoulder dystocia (the shoulders not fitting well through the birth canal) can be a problem.

What you want to avoid is a doctor who uniformly induces all plus-size women. But if your doctor believes that your case is one in which an induction is truly necessary, and if you trust him or her, take the advice.

"At thirty-nine weeks, I was induced because the ultrasound showed low amniotic-fluid levels. Because I was hooked up to the fetal monitor the whole time, I was stuck in bed. This all began Thursday morning. By Sunday around 3 A.M., I was becoming almost hysterical from the confinement. My doctor (who was awful!) was rude to me and my mother and said he didn't believe I would be able to push the baby out. My mother had to force them to check me because they didn't believe me when I said I was ready to push. I ended up pushing her out in twenty minutes."—Heather G.

Anesthesia

Epidurals might not sound terrific right now, but they can be absolute lifesavers for you during labor or birth. Your weight doesn't mean you can't have pain relief during labor, and it doesn't mean it won't be effective. The most-important thing is to be honest with your anesthesiologist about your actual weight. If you feel he or she is insensitive, you can ask for someone else, but be aware that this might mean a longer wait for the pain relief you need.

All epidurals involve placing a catheter into the back. You may have heard of walking epidurals. The strength and type of the epidural depends on the medication that is used. A walking epidural offers pain relief without muscle blockage. An epidural used during a C-section delivers a much-stronger level of medication and pain relief.

A study by the Stanford University School of Medicine looked at placement of epidural catheters (the portion of the epidural that is inserted into your skin). The study recommended that in obese patients, the catheter be inserted at least 4 cm into the epidural space and that patients sit upright or lie on their sides before the catheter is taped to the skin. Doing this reduced the chance the catheter would get moved out of place.

A study by the University of Pittsburgh found that weight is not a factor in a spike in body temperature after receiving an epidural (called epidural fever). There is no correlation between weight and this problem.

A Wake Forest University study found that epidural failure (meaning it doesn't work when inserted) was "significantly more likely" in morbidly obese women than other patients, requiring the catheter to be reinserted. (Note that although it might have had to be reinserted, they always did get it to work.) An Oregon Health & Science University study determined a patient's weight had no impact on the effectiveness of the block provided by an epidural.

An epidural is great for pain relief in labor, and it has the advantage of providing pain relief if you need repair of vaginal lacerations (which can be difficult to repair without anesthesia in an obese or morbidly obese woman because of extra tissue in the area) and allowing for forceps delivery if necessary (also difficult to do without anesthesia). There has been some debate about whether epidurals result in slowed labor. Consensus is that they do not, and, in fact, a recent study indicates that an early epidural (before 4-cm dilation) can actually shorten a woman's labor by ninety minutes. The interpretation of this study is that relaxing without pain will actually help speed the process. This study did not specifically look at plus-size women.

There is some controversy over whether epidurals should be administered to all plus-size women across the board (as opposed to thinner women for whom it is considered just one option available). Some doctors believe it should be done for all plus-size women because if an emergency C-section is needed, pain relief is in place and there will be no need to try to get a spinal done correctly (which can be difficult) or use a general anesthetic. We believe this should remain a decision that is made on an individual basis by considering each woman's circumstances. (See Chapter 14 for more information about the reasons surrounding this controversy.)

Many plus-size women want to have natural labors, and if this is something you desire, you should discuss it with your health-care provider. It is absolutely possible. What is important, though, is to assess your individual circumstances. For example, if there have been no problems with your pregnancy (no medical problems for you or with the baby), you are expecting a normal-sized baby and normal progression of labor (if you've had a normal labor before, this increases your chance of a normal labor again), then an epidural would be unnecessary unless you wanted it for pain relief during labor.

On the other hand, if this is a first pregnancy with poor progression of labor or prolonged ruptured membranes (labor continuing for a long time after the membranes are ruptured, which increases the risk of infection), there is meconium, you have a problem such as hypertension or diabetes, the baby is thought to be large, intubation (inserting a breathing tube for general anesthesia) would be difficult because of your anatomy or weight, problems with placing a spinal or epidural are anticipated (again, because of your anatomy or size), or the monitor has had results that have been of concern, then an epidural would be strongly recommended to you, and you should take that recommendation seriously.

Remember that an epidural is a choice offered to you, and only you can ultimately make the decision to have one. As with all medical procedures, there are always risks involved, and you should ask what these are and what your chances of having a complication are. Your physician and anesthesiologist can offer advice and give opinions based on their experiences, but it is your choice as to what kind of medical care you want to accept.

"The epidural didn't take effect at first, so I had to go through it three times total. The anesthesiologist was not sympathetic. She was short with me and said I was just too fat to stick the needle in far enough."—Julie M.

"The anesthesiologist came in to talk about a spinal. He asked my husband to leave the room, and I insisted he stay. Then he asked me my weight. I had to think a moment (since I was in labor and a bit distracted), and he blew up at me and said, 'See, that's why I wanted him to leave,' as if I was hemming and hawing because I didn't want to say it in front of my husband. It made me really mad because my husband loves me the way I am and is not disgusted by me, and this man acted as if he would be."—Lee T.

"One epidural simply did not work, and they insisted everything was all right. I never had one again."—Amelia M.

"With my third child, an anesthesiologist came in to examine my throat. He said if I needed to be intubated, he might have trouble based on my weight, that overweight patients sometimes had narrow throats. He said he examined all patients more than 280 pounds, just in case. He didn't speak in a discriminatory way, but I was embarrassed."—Margie P.

VBAC: Vaginal Birth after Caesarean Section

The decision about VBAC is one you should make in careful consultation with your OB. VBACs were once thought to be highly safe and effective, but recent research has cast doubt on this for all women. The prevailing consensus is that for a high percentage of women of any size, an elective (meaning it is chosen before labor begins) repeat C-section is safer for both mom and baby than a VBAC, but this appears to be especially true for obese women. What's important to consider, however, is the reason for the first C-section. If you had a C-section for failure to progress in labor, and your second baby seems to be about the same size, it's more likely that your second labor is not going to go anywhere, either, and you'll end up with a C-section. But, if your first baby was a C-section because it was breech, then you might have a better chance of a successful VBAC if this baby is not breech.

The medical preference used to be that it was OK to let a woman try VBAC, and if it didn't work, perform a C-section. However, research now shows that C-sections after failed VBAC attempts have more complications than C-sections performed without the attempt at labor (i.e.

scheduled C-sections). This is true for women of ALL sizes, but because larger women do have a higher rate of slowed labor, which may become failed labor, it's generally believed that an elective C-section is an even safer bet for a plus-size woman than a VBAC attempt. And the research shows that women on the higher end of the plus-size group spectrum tend to have greater difficulties after VBACs. A University of Florida study found that when very obese women had VBACs, 25 percent developed infections after the birth, whereas only 8 percent of the obese women who had C-sections did. The risk for overweight or mildly obese women appears to be lower.

"I didn't even try VBAC. My doctor said it was likely I was going to need a C-section anyhow, so why go through labor again?"—Brenda Z.

"After my C-section, I was not sure I'd ever want another child. The delivery and recovery were so hard compared to vaginal (how I had my first child). Time passed, though, and we decided to have another baby. At the first doctor visit, I asked about VBAC and asked for resources as well as her personal experience. The doctor had some printed information for me, but not anything really useful. She felt that if the pregnancy went well and the baby's weight remained within normal limits I had a strong chance of a successful VBAC. I had this discussion with each of the four doctors as my visits came up. They all felt comfortable with VBAC. They did review the risks, but also the benefits of vaginal versus C-section. No one tried to discourage me, but they all stressed the fact that they would not let the labor become prolonged (like it did with my C-section baby). At the first sign of fetal distress, they would insist on a C-section. Close to delivery, I had to sign some forms stating I understood the risks involved with VBAC and gave the doctors the right to move to a C-section in the event of my health or the baby's being at risk. The doctors felt that I would stand a better chance of VBAC if the baby was smaller than the C-section baby. Since the baby was growing fast, they recommended induction at thirty-eight weeks if I had not delivered on my own. The induction was dreadful, and the contractions so much more intense than the other two natural labors I experienced. I was able to deliver vaginally, but in the process ripped some of the old scar tissue from the C-section, which resulted in an umbilical hernia for which I've had two surgeries."—Beth T.

14

C-sections

*I*f you have to have a C-section, the most-important thing to remember is that you are still having a baby, and that is all that matters. Having a C-section doesn't make you less of a mom or mean you failed in any way. In fact, there are probably some women with long, painful labors who will envy you. Lots and lots of women have C-sections (about 25 percent of all births are performed this way), so you're not alone. The goal of your whole pregnancy is a healthy baby. If your doctor says the best way to get there is to have a C-section, then do it happily. No, it's not fun, but it's not unbearable either. It's something you can definitely get through if it means a healthy baby.

C-section Likelihood

Case Western Reserve University did a study recently and found that 10.4 percent of "overweight" women who had not previously had a C-section needed one, as well as 13.8 percent of "obese" women, compared with 7.7 percent of "normal" women. The study also considered preexisting diabetes and gestational diabetes and found that weight by itself is a separate risk factor (previous studies were questioned because they didn't consider the impact diabetes may have had on the results).

Another study showed that women (presumably of average size) who gain more than the recommended twenty-five to thirty-five pounds in pregnancy are more likely to have C-sections. The study did not specifically consider if C-sections are also more likely when larger women gain more than the recommended amount of weight.

A C-section is probably not your ideal birth, but if you have one, you need to know what to expect and how to cope. Your weight does not mean that a C-section will be more complicated or last longer.

One reason often cited for the high rate of C-sections in plus-size women is that larger women often have larger babies, although this is not always the case. If you have a C-section and your baby turns out to be average or small, it doesn't mean you or your doctor made a mistake. (See Chapter 16 for more information about large babies and C-sections.) Some labors just don't progress, and some babies just won't come out on their own—it's not your fault. C-sections are also common in larger women because of a higher rate of gestational diabetes. But big babies and diabetes are not always the reason. It is theorized that increased body fat in the pelvic area may compress the bony pelvis and make the dimensions of it smaller, making it harder to deliver the baby.

C-sections are something doctors, and most patients, want to avoid because of the increased risk to the mother, the longer recovery time, and the discomfort. But when a baby is too large or labor is not progressing, they can provide a happy ending for all involved. If you're concerned about C-sections, take a childbirth preparation class or a vaginal birth after Caesarean class if you've had a previous C-section. Talk with your health-care provider about the size and position of your baby. Find out what your health-care provider's C-section rate is. Midwife practices usually have lower C-section rates, but this may be because women at higher risk of C-sections opt to see obstetricians instead.

If you have a C-section, it's important that it be done by an obstetrician and that the obstetrician is experienced in performing C-sections on plus-size women, so that any risks and complications can be minimized. Remember, a C-section is not the end of the world and is simply another method of giving birth.

Some doulas and midwives interviewed for this book have reported hearing doctors place bets on how far their larger patients will progress in labor before needing a C-section. This is insensitive and rude (and we hope not widespread). Let's hope that you have been able to locate a size-friendly health-care provider for your pregnancy, and this will not be a problem for you.

"I had a C-section with my twins, and I knew, because of my high blood pressure, that's probably what it would be. I have to say, it wasn't bad. The recovery time was a little more difficult, but not as bad as I thought."—Beth U.

"Just tell yourself, if it takes a C-section, that's OK . . . you did it! You nourished a wonderful baby inside of you for nine months. It's a miracle, and who cares how the baby has to come out."—Peggy M.

"Second time around I knew I was having a big baby, and because of that, a Caesarean was scheduled to prevent a recurrence of an incident during the first birth when my daughter was stuck and needed to be forcibly pulled out during a vaginal delivery."—Sharon L.

Pain Relief for C-sections

There is controversy about whether spinals or epidurals are better for C-sections involving plus-size women. Some doctors feel that an epidural is the best answer because it can be given during labor and then just kept in. When an epidural is given during labor, there is no rush to insert it, as there would be in giving a spinal in an emergency C-section situation.

An emergency C-section is one that occurs when the baby is in distress, the mother is bleeding heavily (which can indicate placenta abruption or placenta previa), or the fetal-monitor results are of immediate concern. In an emergency, the medical team needs to perform an immediate spinal or use general anesthesia. Many women have nonemergency C-sections after going through labor. These C-sections happen when there is failure to progress in labor, but there is no immediate danger to the mom or baby. In this situation, there is time to place a spinal.

The epidural can be used for pain relief during labor, and then if an emergency C-section is needed, it is just kept in, medication levels are increased, and it's used to provide pain relief during the surgery. The problem with this approach is that epidurals can provide patchy pain relief—you may not get complete and thorough pain blockage. And during a surgery, this is a problem. The other problem is that because it's just easier to give an epidural during labor, some physicians are recommending epidurals for all plus-size patients when they get to the hospital whether they need it or not. A 1999 Duke University study concluded that obese moms are twice as likely to have a C-section. Based on this study, Duke obstetric anesthesiologists now recommend that all obese women be given epidurals in case an emergency C-section becomes necessary. Some doctors agree with this approach, while others think it may be a rush to judgment. Plus-size women should be encouraged to consider an epidural if they want pain relief and have the benefits of it explained to them.

It's not just plus-size moms that use epidurals for pain relief in a C-section. Dr. Bruce D. Rodgers, coauthor of this book, finds that of the total C-sections at his hospital, half are epidural and half spinal. Epidurals for C-sections are not something just being used for plus-size women in his experience.

If you're in labor and don't have an epidural and for some reason need an emergency C-section, but the anesthesiologist can't do it successfully in time, you're going to end up with general anesthesia, which has even higher risks. Obese women are difficult to intubate, and emergency intubation is always dangerous in a pregnant woman, regardless of size.

Some doctors still prefer spinals for C-sections. A spinal works immediately, while an epidural takes ten to fifteen minutes to take effect. A spinal provides complete pain relief. However, the spinal has the disadvantage of being a one-shot deal—you can't add to it in the middle of surgery. (The catheter is not left in as it is with an epidural—the anesthesia is injected into the spine using a needle and it is then removed.) If the surgery goes longer than expected and it begins to wear off, you would require general anesthesia. An increased length of surgery is usually a concern only for morbidly obese women. A spinal also has a higher risk of causing hypotension (low blood pressure) than an epidural, which can result in decreased blood flow to the uterus causing problems for the baby. Some studies have shown lower Apgar scores (a scoring system used after birth that evaluates the baby) and lower cord pH values (indicating some oxygen deprivation to the baby) from spinals.

In obese and morbidly obese women, spinal and epidural anesthesia is more difficult to administer, may require multiple attempts, and may take more time to put in place. The reason is that it may be harder for the anesthesiologist to find the right spot if there is a lot of tissue in that area.

Physicians also report having more difficulty placing the breathing tube in obese moms when general anesthesia is used. When you are in the hospital, a nurse or anesthesiologist may ask to look down your throat to see if there is a clear path.

Since large women have a higher chance of needing a regular or emergency C-section and, because of their weight, have a greater chance of complications from general anesthesia (usually only done for

Caesareans in extreme emergencies or when the spinal/epidural fails), most doctors believe that serious consideration should be given to offering obese women an elective epidural, usually around 4 cm dilation.

The best approach to making a decision about anesthesia is to see the anesthesiologist early in labor to map out a plan and to decide what the best strategy for anesthesia would be if a C-section is needed. You also need to talk to your OB about this during your pregnancy so you have some time to think about it and absorb his or her advice. If this is your first baby, you're probably not planning on it being a C-section (although more and more women do make that choice), but it's important to realize that a C-section is a possibility. If you ignore it, you could end up in a situation where you have to make a decision without a lot of knowledge. It's best to think about the options now and learn about the reasoning behind the recommendations, so you can make an educated choice if necessary.

"I had a spinal. My doctor told me she had an epidural for hers, and she felt everything on the left side. I didn't have any problems with it."—Lee T.

"The labor was very long. I was completely dilated and effaced, but no amount of pushing could get him delivered. The doctor considered he might be breech, but an ultrasound ruled that out. He was facing upward, toward the ceiling, which combined with his large head, made delivery very hard. During the transition phase of labor, I requested the epidural. After I had been dilated and pushing four-plus hours, it was the doctor's recommendation that we go for a C-section. The baby's heartbeat had been dropping during the hard contractions and during pushing, we lost it altogether sometimes. The doctor explained the risks of continued vaginal attempts versus the risks of a C-section. While explaining, we lost the heartbeat again, and even with an internal monitor, they could not get a heartbeat. It became an emergency, and I was taken right to the operating room. They did not ask about the spinal, they just told me that the epidural would not be enough and that I had to have the spinal. Once in the operating room, they injected the spinal and immediately prepped me for the C-section. I'm not sure how fast the spinal works, but thankfully, I did not feel it when they operated."—Beth T.

"I had an epidural with my first. We were trying for a natural birth, but he got hung up breech in my ribs and needed forceps to get him out in the section. I loved the epidural. It was great, complete coverage. I threw up afterward, though. With my second, I had a spinal. That made me anxious. My sister had a spinal headache after hers. I didn't though. But I tend to be phobic about not feeling myself breathe, so I was really worried about that part. It was OK though, my chest didn't go so numb as the rest of me. I think that they are doing a spinal for my third. To be honest, I think it seems to be hospital policy that sections are done with a spinal. If I had a choice, I'd go with the epidural. The person administering it was wonderful, and when they asked me in surgery if I could feel anything (and I did a lot), they just turned it up until I didn't feel anything at all."—Cheryl H

Incisions

There are two types of incisions in every C-section: the incision made in the skin (abdominal incision) and the incision made in the womb (uterine incision). The horizontal abdominal incision used for most C-sections is known medically as a Pfannensteil incision (named after the surgeon who invented it), and is commonly referred to as a "bikini cut" (since most two-piece bathing suits would hide the incision). The uterine incision most commonly used is also horizontal and is made in the lower part of the uterus just beneath the bikini cut skin incision. This uterine incision is referred to medically as a low segment transverse C-section (LFTCS). A horizontal incision in both the abdomen and uterus are standard practice for most C-sections performed at term (full gestational age).

Vertical incisions high on the uterus are called classical C-sections (since this is the way all Cesareans were performed many decades ago). These are performed only for special circumstances, since they don't heal as well and are more prone to rupture in future pregnancies.

There is debate over what type of abdominal incision is best for plus-size women. The common choices are the bikini cut or vertical skin incision (done on the lower abdomen in an up-and-down direction).

The bikini cut is made just above the pubic bone. The problem in plus-size women is this incision is at the very bottom of the tummy area, and you may have a tummy that sags or hangs over a bit (called a pannus). The incision may be covered by this, stay damp, and not get very good airflow, leading to possible bacteria growth. The weight of your stomach may also pull on the incision, causing problems with the staples staying in. Because of this, the low-abdominal vertical skin incision is sometimes advocated for obese women, especially morbidly obese women. But these vertical incisions are less cosmetically appealing, more painful, and more predisposed to wound disruption. You should talk to your OB about the type of incision that would be recommended for you.

C-section Complications

If you have a C-section, you should know that larger women can have more complications after the surgery than smaller women. We're going to examine some of these complications so you understand what they are and how they are treated. The good news is that these types of complications are highly preventable and very treatable if they do occur. Don't get upset thinking that they're going to happen to you or that they are horrible, irreversible problems. Remember, if you have a C-section, the most important thing is that you've delivered a healthy and wonderful baby. Your body needs time to heal and recover from the surgery and if you have a few bumps along the road, try not to worry.

Blood Clots

There are two kinds of thromboembolic events (blood-clotting problems). Deep vein thrombosis (DVT) is a blood clot in the veins of the leg or pelvis. Pulmonary embolism is when a blood clot from a leg or pelvic vein breaks off and moves to an artery in a lung. It sounds scary, but it can be prevented.

The combination of obesity, pregnancy, and C-section increases the risk of thromboembolic events after delivery. The risk is greater if the woman smokes, is older than thirty-five, has varicose veins, or if the C-section is an emergency. There are several types of prevention that will effectively minimize your risks. One method is to receive a small dose of Heparin (a blood thinner) just before surgery. The dose is very small and does not increase the risk of bleeding during surgery. Heparin must be given after the epidural catheter is inserted and often requires that the removal of the epidural catheter be delayed until after the surgery. Another option is a dose of Heparin after delivery. There is some evidence that an epidural reduces the risk of DVT.

The safest and most-common prevention method, however, is the use of what are called sequential or intermittent pneumatic compression devices, which look like blood-pressure cuffs that are put on each of your calves prior to surgery. They inflate and deflate, and they're left on until you're up and walking. All plus-size women who have C-sections should have these. Once you're mobile, you'll be given white compression stockings that go over your calves, called antiembolism stockings, which you'll be asked to wear while you're in the hospital recovering. Getting on your feet and walking as soon as possible is important, within twelve to eighteen hours after surgery. The risk of DVT is highest after delivery and lasts up to six weeks postpartum, but these treatments can significantly reduce the risk. If you experience significant leg swelling, leg pain, chest pain, or shortness of breath anytime after delivery, you should get in touch with your doctor immediately.

"I remember those leg-cuff things. It felt like getting your blood pressure taken. Then I had these silly looking knee-highs that had no toes."—Kathleen J.

Incision Problems
Incision infections are relatively high after C-sections no matter a woman's size. They are even more likely when they are performed for

emergencies, after labor or after prolonged ruptured membranes. They are also more likely in plus-size women. The infections can be in the part of the uterus that was cut or in the surrounding tissue in the abdomen. Preventative antibiotics should be given since this reduces the risk of both types of infection. They can be given prior to the surgery or just after the baby is delivered when the umbilical cord is clamped. Doing so after the delivery works just as well and prevents the baby from being exposed to the antibiotic. Irrigation (rinsing) of the subcutaneous tissue (fat or adipose tissue) just before the wound is closed is also highly effective. Your surgeon should carefully check and cauterize (use a special instrument to stop bleeding) all bleeding areas.

Morbidly obese women should have sutures (stitches) placed in the fat tissue so there is no space in the fat under the skin (which can lead to infection). A pressure dressing (special adhesive tape over the wound dressing), which puts pressure on the tissue, causes any bleeding or oozing from capillaries to stop, preventing infection. For morbidly obese women, a subcutaneous drain can be used, which reduces complications. The drains are plastic tubes connected to a small plastic container with suction. The part of the drain inside the incision allows blood and fluid to be sucked out. Drains are lightweight, small, and easy to remove. Removal is done at the bedside, usually on the second day after surgery.

A recent study showed that careful wound care of the horizontal bikini skin incision in plus-size women can prevent wound infections. In very obese women, the bikini cut may not be an option purely due to inability to access the lower abdomen under the pannus. However, mildly obese women and overweight women can usually have a bikini incision as long as they have careful wound care. If you think a C-section is an option for you, talk to your OB about incision types beforehand.

"Some of my staples pulled out when I was in the shower at the hospital. I didn't real-ize that was what had happened. I remember tipping back to wash my hair and feel-ing a pulling sensation, and I guess that's when it happened. They noticed it the next day and had to restaple it. It was pretty rough. They shot me up with drugs and did it in my hospital room. I went home with staples in. Not fun, but it didn't get infected or anything, fortunately. The doctor told me that with my next [child], she is going to cut out some of the scar tissue during the surgery."—Kathleen J.

"With my first C-section, I was knocked out and had an extra surgery to remove all the fat from my bellybutton down (it's called a panniculectomy). This was to help me out and to help with infection after the C-section. It helped a lot, but with both, it took awhile men-tally to look at it."—Jennifer H.

C-section Postpartum Care

Your incision is going to be really sore, and so is your entire abdomen. Your first reaction will probably be to just not touch it and avoid letting other people touch or look at it. It's really crucial, though, that you let the nurses examine your incision at least once a day. If you need cushion-ing or dressing, a clean sanitary pad can be placed over the incision. But if you do this, try to lie down, pull up your gown, and gently press any hanging tummy areas up for a few minutes a few times a day to let some air get on the incision. Your health-care provider may tell you to rinse the area with a mixture of water and hydrogen peroxide once or twice a day. Careful incision care can prevent infections, so it's important to do this as directed. If you notice any redness or have any discharge from the inci-sion, let your health-care provider know immediately.

It's essential that you get up and move around after the surgery to avoid blood clots and breathing problems, as discussed earlier in the chapter. It's not fun, but it is important. Just take it slow, and make sure there is someone there to help you. Moving around will also help you pass gas, and the nurses won't let you eat until you pass gas, so use that as your incentive.

Talk to your doctor about what restrictions to follow once you're home, such as not climbing stairs or lifting heavy things for a certain period of time. Remember that you're going to be just plain sore for a while. Getting up out of bed can be really painful (since you use your abdominal muscles to pull your body up), so using pillows to prop yourself up before you try can help. You could place a chair next to the bed, hold on to that, and use it to pull yourself up by your arms. You can also roll onto your side, put your legs over the side of the bed, and then slowly push yourself up using the strength of your arms.

You should talk to your health-care provider about exercises to regain abdominal muscle control. Many larger women later find that they experience back problems, which could have been avoided if they had regained strength in their abdominal muscles after a C-section.

Breastfeeding in the traditional position may be uncomfortable after a C-section, so be sure to see a lactation consultant. Be aware that your milk may take longer to come in after a C-section. It will come in eventually, so don't worry that you won't have any.

The most important thing to do after a C-section is just take care of yourself. You need time to rest and recuperate. Yes, you want to spend time with your baby and you have a home to take care of, but you must make time to rest. Everything else in life can wait. The better you care for yourself in the first few weeks, the better you'll feel in the coming months.

Don't worry about what your body looks like after the surgery. The incision is going to look, well, like an incision. It will take a while to heal completely. You may feel bloated, puffy, sore, and somehow just weird in the days and weeks afterward. Your body needs time to heal, and the way it looks is completely normal. Even thin women who have C-sections feel and look horrible for weeks. It's not you, and it's not your size. You've had major surgery. Give it some time.

"Recovery wasn't bad while on pain meds in the hospital. The trick is to get up often and get your bowels moving so you can get home."—Cheryl H.

"They assumed I would not heal as well as a thinner person. I surprised my doctor and healed 'better than anyone he has ever seen,' in his words."—Julie M.

"I had severe postpartum infection due to, as my doctor put it, 'fat doesn't heal well.' The large hanging belly apparently caused it. I was told to roll up a cloth under the belly so the air would hit the incision. Wrong. I advise others to use a sterile dressing and be on the lookout for any sign of infection."—Peggy M.

"I just used a large pad over the six-inch drain, stapled incision. When they asked me to cough, I would hold a pillow over it and push a little. It did fine. Try and keep your incision clean to prevent infections under the belly apron of fat."—Jen R.

With my second section, I had a hard time seeing the incision to keep it clean, so that was uncomfortable."—Angie G.

15

Leaky Watermelons and Sour Milk:
Nursing as a Plus-Size Mom

The American Academy of Pediatrics recommends that all babies be breast fed for the first year (and exclusively breast-fed for the first six months), if possible. Breastfeeding has been shown to prevent illness, increase IQ, reduce food allergies, improve bonding, and decrease the likelihood that a child will be over-weight. If you can't or don't want to breast feed, don't despair. Bottle-fed babies are happy, healthy, and intelligent, too, and what really matters is that you feel comfortable with your feeding choice. This chapter will focus on breastfeeding concerns, but also has some information about choosing not to breast feed and stories from moms who have made this decision.

Loving Your Larger Breasts

You may not be thrilled to be done with pregnancy and still have big, uncomfortable breasts. You might find your breasts to be in the way, annoying, leaky, or just too big. Remind yourself that your breasts are providing complete and perfect nutrition for your baby. They are amazing food factories, creating full-course, liquid meals to satisfy your baby's every need.

Your baby certainly doesn't care what size your breasts are and is always going to be happy to latch on and feed. Keeping in mind that your breasts are performing an important and difficult job will help you appreciate them even more. And it's not forever—just until you decide you're done nursing.

"Love your big breasts! Revel in the beauty of nursing! Remember that your baby adores you no matter what size you are."—Amelia M.

Breastfeeding Success

Your body is ready to begin feeding your baby soon after he or she is born. However, some moms have difficulty with breastfeeding, and some of these problems are common in plus-size women. Women of all shapes and sizes can experience difficulty with nursing, and it's a good idea to understand what the research says so you understand the reasons for it.

Plus-size moms can sometimes have difficulty with milk supply. A study published in the journal *Pediatrics* found that overweight moms are 2.5 times less successful in beginning breastfeeding than other women, and obese moms are 3.6 times less successful. Let's put these numbers in perspective though. According to a national study done by Ross Products (a formula company), in 2000, 68.4 percent of all women breast fed in the hospital, and 31.4 percent were still breastfeeding at six months.

Larger women produce less prolactin, a hormone made by the pituitary gland that stimulates breast-milk production. In the study above, overweight and obese women produced dramatically less prolactin forty-eight hours after the birth, but the levels were closer to normal seven days after birth (although still slightly lower).

During pregnancy, progesterone levels are very high. After delivery, the progesterone level drops and is the trigger for milk secretion. Nursing then produces prolactin, which is important for continued milk production. Another study in *Pediatrics* showed that the problem with obese women was not higher progesterone levels (they theorized that since progesterone is concentrated in fat tissue obese women may have elevated progesterone levels released from fat which inhibits milk secretion), but a diminished prolactin response to nursing. The good news is that prolactin is not as important for breastfeeding after seven days. They found that most obese women who give up on breastfeeding do so in the first week. Therefore, if you stick with it for more than a week, you are more likely to be successful. That first week may be rocky, so plan ahead, and know you may need support from a lactation consultant.

Keep in mind that these studies did not actually measure milk supply and only tracked the number of women who were successful with breastfeeding.

There is also some evidence that Polycystic Ovarian Syndrome (see Chapter 7 for more information) may have a connection to low milk supply. If you have this, you should talk to your doctor. It has been estimated that up to 20 percent of PCOS patients will encounter difficulty breastfeeding. It's not clear if it's weight or metabolic problems (women with gestational diabetes have similar problems to women with PCOS and insulin resistance is common to both conditions) that cause the problem. It's probably a combination of many factors. There is very little research available about PCOS and breastfeeding. The good news is that most PCOS patients will do just fine breastfeeding. If you have PCOS, it is a good idea to talk to your health-care provider about breastfeeding during your pregnancy.

A study in the *Journal of Human Lactation* in 2004 found that women with a higher body mass tend to have their milk come in later (over seventy-two hours after the birth) than thinner women (who had milk come in within seventy-two hours). This study does not mean plus-size moms can't breast feed, but it can mean it might naturally take longer for your milk to come in. If this happens, you should talk to your child's health-care providers about whether you need to supplement with formula in the beginning.

A study in the October 2000 issue of the *Journal of Paediatrics and Child Health* showed that among women with a body mass index of 20 to 25, 89.2 percent began breastfeeding, while among women with a BMI of more than 30, 82.3 percent began breastfeeding. The study did not address the kind of care and support the women received or what level of encouragement they got with regard to breastfeeding, nor did it consider all the other lifestyle and health factors that can influence a woman's decision to breast feed. This study does show that plus-size moms are less likely to try breastfeeding. If breastfeeding is something you want to try, you shouldn't let anyone discourage you or make you feel inadequate.

Another related study looked at average-weight women who gained twenty-four to thirty-five pounds during pregnancy and found that they were 74 percent more likely to be unsuccessful with breastfeeding, concluding that excessive weight gain during pregnancy may affect breastfeeding success. However, this study looked at average women who gained more than the recommended weight during pregnancy and did not look at larger-sized women at all. It's probably a good assumption that gaining too much weight during pregnancy will impact breastfeeding success for any woman.

All of this evidence might lead some professionals to conclude that larger women just can't be successful with breastfeeding. Be aware that you might be facing prejudice and lack of support from the beginning. If you're serious about breastfeeding, don't stop trying, and be sure to ask for help if you need it.

The American Academy of Family Physicians says that the keys to successful breastfeeding include:

- Beginning as soon as possible after birth
- Frequent feedings (eight to twelve times a day in the first twelve weeks)
- Proper latch (making sure the baby's mouth holds the nipple the right way)
- Correct positioning (holding the baby the right way)
- Drinking enough fluids
- Making sure the baby is swallowing and not just sucking
- Talk to your lactation consultant for more specific information and counseling

"I have PCOS and IGT (insufficient glandular tissue) and had complete milk supply failure with my first daughter. During my second pregnancy, I actually grew breast tissue and was able to have a successful breastfeeding relationship with my second daughter."—Andrea H.

"I wasn't able to breastfeed. My milk never came in, and one nurse did blame it on my weight. Something about my breasts being more than two inches apart and the fact that they never changed much or got bigger during my pregnancy and some other things. I tried to feed her for a month supplementing with formula, but she wasn't gaining any weight, so I gave up and switched to formula. Of all the problems I thought I was to encounter getting pregnant, being pregnant, and giving birth, it never occurred to me that I wouldn't be able to breastfeed. I spent weeks crying and beating myself up over this. But I came to realize I have a happy, healthy baby, and that's the most important thing."—Tammy M.

"Drink lots of water, but limit it after 5 P.M. so that you're not up all night going to the bathroom."—Amelia M.

Choosing Not to Breastfeed

Some women feel bullied into breastfeeding. It's a personal choice, though, and if breastfeeding doesn't work for you, you don't want to try it, or you hate it, you are still a good mother who will be able to raise a healthy and happy child. Your child needs your love more than anything, and if you can provide that, you've succeeded as a mom. Talk to your pediatrician about formula options if breastfeeding isn't going to be part of your plan. Formula provides excellent nutrition, and your baby is going to grow up perfectly fine drinking it. Carrying around guilt or worry about formula-feeding is just going to make you, and by association, your baby, miserable. Moms who use formula are good moms, too.

"Breastfeeding has been full of guilt for me. It's uncomfortable, and heavy breasts point down, plus with Caesareans, it has been hard. I pumped with my first baby for around six weeks and with the second one only breast-fed around a week or so. Breastfeeding brought out so many emotions for me. It's like my hormones were on a rampage, and I cried every time I had to do it. So much pressure and I was never sure if it was enough for the baby. Perhaps I should have kept it up, but I felt drained and too emotional to continue. This brought on so much guilt. What kind of a mother thinks more of herself than her baby's well-being? We found formula with breast-milk ingredients and used the Good Starts, so I began to feel better."—Cheryl H.

"I really hated pumping breast milk every two hours, as my breasts hurt. They augmented my breast milk in the NICU with formula. After six months of torture pumping breast milk, my doctor advised [me to] stop. I believe that mothers who feed formula, which was nearly every mother in the NICU, need to be supported, as well as breastfeeding mothers. There's a huge breastfeeding lobby in this country who are fanatical about breastfeeding and trying to force their ideas and beliefs off on every mother out there, in a fascist manner that is disgusting and wrong. Formula-feeding is a legitimate option."—DeAnn R.

"Breastfeeding didn't work for me. I did it for three months. I had a hard time, and I think a lot of it was because my breasts were so big."—Deb P.

Getting Help

Patricia Lindsey-Salvo, R.N., coordinator of the Breastfeeding Center of Manhattan, has given thought to the statistics and problems facing breastfeeding plus-size moms and still concludes it is an important option to try if you can. "breastfeeding decreases an infant's risk of obesity, diabetes, and cardiovascular disease. We live in a society that has lost the art of breastfeeding, and mothers are often given very bad advice. Some health professionals are still not practicing using evidence-based information."

Her best advice if you want to breast feed is "See a lactation consultant. I would suggest that all moms [attend] a prenatal evidence-based breastfeeding class so that they are fueled with correct information. Nothing sabotages breastfeeding more than incorrect myths."

Don't give up—be committed to it. Work with a board-certified lactation consultant—there will be one at the hospital at which you deliver at and your pediatrician should have one on staff or at least be able to refer you to one.

Lindsey-Salvo encourages plus-size moms to breast feed despite the difficulties they may face. "We have many larger women successful at breastfeeding. Poor positioning and not enough breastfeeding are reasons for decreased milk supply. The most-prevalent reason is not enough breastfeeding or doing both bottle and breast. When [plus-size moms in our program] left the hospital exclusively breastfeeding, six months later, 57 percent are still breastfeeding. Of those who left doing both, only 17 percent were still breastfeeding at six months."

Lindsey-Salvo strongly suggests that you continue to seek help from a lactation consultant after the baby is born, "A complete assessment needs to be made. Latch checks are the most important. A baby can look like it is breastfeeding, but only be nipple-feeding. There is no milk in the nipple. Sore nipples, a hungry baby, and decreased milk supply are all results of a poor latch."

La Leche League is especially tuned into the breastfeeding concerns of women with large breasts. You can read articles about breastfeeding with large breasts online at: *www.lalecheleague.org/llleaderweb/LV/ LVMayJun89p35.html* and *www.lalecheleague.org/llleaderweb/LV/LVAugSep 00p63.html*. If these links do not work, access the home page at *www.lalecheleague.org*, and contact the Webmaster asking where to find the *Leaven* Tips from Leaders from May–June 1989 and August–September 2000. Additionally, La Leche League has approximately one hundred leaders who specialize in large breasts. To contact one, go to *www.laleacheleague.org*, and use the online help form. La Leche recommends that women attend at least four local meetings to obtain information and support before they give birth. If you have smaller breasts (many plus-size women are not a D cup!) you can still seek help—La Leche is dedicated to breastfeeding success for all women, regardless of breast size or weight. If you are experiencing problems with breastfeeding, another resource is the Yahoo group Mothers Overcoming Breastfeeding Issues (MOBI) at *http://health.groups.yahoo.com/group/MOBI/*.

Andrea Henderson, a birth doula in New Mexico, says, "Do not let anyone tell you your breasts or nipples are too big. They might be big, but a lactation consultant can help with those issues. I encourage all my clients to see the hospital lactation consultant before leaving the hospital. Oftentimes, the lactation consultant can spot potential problems that might not become a full-blown issue until mother and baby are home for a few days." She also points out that establishing a relationship with the consultant while in the hospital will make you feel more comfortable if you need to call her once you're home.

If you have very large breasts, latching on may prove to be your biggest hurdle to breastfeeding success. Seeing a lactation consultant (both in the hospital and after you leave) can help you learn strategies to get your baby to latch on correctly.

The key to successful breastfeeding is seeking out information and support when you run into a problem. Don't feel as if your size or body shape automatically means breastfeeding will not be easy for you, and don't assume that professionals won't know how to help you or have experience working with plus-size moms. There are a lot of professionals who feel very passionately about breastfeeding for all women, and if you need help, they are there for you.

> "I had a difficult time breastfeeding my boys due to a possible low milk supply. I later found out that I had severe hypothyroidism that could have contributed to my low supply, as well as my difficulty losing weight."—Dana C.
>
> "This research really hit home for me. My son weighed eight pounds, fourteen ounces at birth, but by the time he was nine months old, he was in the bottom 20 percent for weight, and by the time he was a year, he was in the bottom 15 percent (he later rebounded). We have big kids, so this was very concerning to us. I am now wondering if I had low milk supply. The pediatrician never suggested that as a possibility, and I feel sick to think that he might not have been getting enough. I'm pregnant now, and I have to say this makes me feel like supplementing with formula might not be so completely evil."—Lee T.

Help with Milk Supply

Breast growth during pregnancy is the first key to milk supply. Most women grow a cup size and notice changes in areola coloring and increased prominence of veins in the breasts. If you don't experience any changes like this during pregnancy, talk to your health-care provider. Once the baby is born, work with a lactation consultant. If your consultant feels that you are having milk-supply problems, there are solutions. Increasing the amount of breastfeeding or pumping can help to stimulate production. Drinking a lot of water can also help. If you have sore nipples, talk to your lactation consultant about home remedies (like placing cold cabbage leaves in your bra), as well as over-the-counter creams (such as Lansinoh).

Galactagogues are drugs that aid in lactation, usually by increasing milk supply. The two most common prescription galactatogues are metoclopramide (Reglan) and domperidone (Motilium). They work by increasing prolactin levels. Domperidone is not available in the U.S. Reglan causes postpartum depression in some women and may have other side effects. Overall, though, it has a good track record for effectiveness and safety for both mother and baby (but use should be closely monitored for signs of depression). There are also some herbal galactagogues. Most lactation specialists feel that galactagogues should be used only as a last resort and only after all conservative measures have been tried, including consultation with a certified lactation consultant. Extreme care should be used in taking herbal galactoagogues, and it's wise to consult with a health-care professional and your pediatrician before trying any.

Herbal remedies are not always regulated by the FDA for purity. It's important to be cautious when using them. Some may be potentially dangerous for the mother and/or baby. Fenugreek was studied and did not appear to be harmful, but there was no control group and no convincing evidence of its effectiveness.

Metformin (Glucophage) is another drug that can be a help in increasing milk supply. Metformin is used to treat type 2 diabetes. It has gained recognition lately as an effective treatment for infertility and recurrent miscarriage in women with PCOS. Because of this, and because PCOS patients may experience lactation failure, it may be useful as a treatment for lactation failure in these patients. There are no well-known studies to support this, however. Glucophage is considered safe for women with diabetes who are breastfeeding since little of the drug gets into the breast milk. If a PCOS woman is having lactation failure, and all other traditional methods have failed, it may be an option to try this, but only under the supervision of a health-care professional and with the consent of the baby's pediatrician.

It's important to be aware of medications and substances that can inhibit lactation. Smoking inhibits lactation. In addition, ergot-alkaloid drugs, such as Methergine (sometimes used after delivery to stop uterine bleeding), can inhibit milk supply. Pseudoephedrine and ephedrine (found in over-the-counter cold and allergy medication) may inhibit lactation, as well.

If you have diabetes, you may experience a delay in your milk coming in. Nurse (or pump) as soon as possible, and as often as possible, to stimulate the supply. The key to being successful with breastfeeding is not to give up, even if you encounter early problems. It can be really difficult to keep pumping and keep nursing when there's nothing coming out. You feel like a failure, you're worried the baby is going to starve, the pumping may be uncomfortable, and on top of that, you're coping with the huge emotional changes that come when you have a newborn. You feel like a complete wreck. Keeping at something that makes you feel like a failure can be a miserable experience. If you really want to do it, remind yourself that you're just having some temporary problems. Get a lactation consultant to talk you through everything, and rely on her for support. Remember, studies show that things should get better after the first week. If you can hang on that long, things might work out. If you finally decide you can't deal with it, that's OK, too.

Comfortable Nursing Positions

Lindsey-Salvo, R.N., recognizes that larger moms sometimes have difficulty figuring out breastfeeding positions that will work. "Large-breasted women do have to adjust positioning for comfort and the proper latch-on. The football hold works well for many large-breasted women. Side-by-side nursing on a bed may also work well and provide a comfortable position."

Some women find that sitting cross-legged on the floor and putting several pillows next to their thigh can provide a comfortable way to support the baby while using the football hold. It can be awkward in a chair if you don't have a lot of space next to you. You can also use nursing pillows to help support the baby in any position you are using. You may get a tired arm or hand from constant feeding, so use pillows to help make things more comfortable.

It's important to support your breast while the baby is nursing. Use the C hold, with your thumb on one side and your fingers on the other and your breast supported in the palm of your hand. If your hand or arm gets tired, you might try rolling up a small towel and placing it under the breast to help hold it up. Lying on your side may eliminate the need to hold up your breast during nursing and give your hands a rest.

"The football hold is sometimes easier."—Rachel G.

"I often found that having a pillow for my little boy to lie on was easier for me. When I was learning, I had him at my side, rather than across my lap. It seemed to help since most of my lap tended to get taken up by stomach."—Amanda F.

"The best advice I ever got: lay down! All nursing mothers in nature (animals) nurse in the position they sleep. Period. It's tough to compare yourself with a dog or cat, I know, but it's natural. Lie on your side with baby on his/her side facing you. This automatically puts baby in the perfect position for nursing (ear-shoulder-hip-knees aligned) so that he latches on correctly and you don't get sore nipples. You are forced to rest and relax, which makes the milk flow better."—Vanessa R.

"I hated breastfeeding because my breasts always seemed to cover the baby's whole face. I asked a nurse about this, and she said that a baby won't let herself suffocate. She'll pull away if she needs air."—Ali S.

"I still get jealous of perky-breasted moms who can lift a shirt and pop the baby on. My south-pointing nipples make this impossible. The hardest time is the first couple of months when my breast is larger than the baby. I think it is overwhelming to the baby, and I have to support my breast all the time. Now, as I nurse my nine-month-old, she can find my nipple and latch on easily—I no longer need to support my breast. My stomach acts as a ledge—

almost helpful. When I nurse in public, I keep most of the weight of my breast in my bra so my nipple is upturned. This helps with positioning in the sling for nursing."—Margie P.

Finding Nursing Bras, Clothing, Baby Carriers, and Slings

As if breastfeeding isn't difficult enough, finding nursing bras and equipment can seem like an impossible task for plus-size women.

Look for cotton bras (cotton will breathe and keep your nipples from getting sore) without underwires (which can cause plugged ducts) when shopping for a nursing bra. You may also want to look for flaps that have large overlap (so you don't have your breast peeking out around the edges of the flaps) and hooks that are easy to undo and do back up with one hand.

If you're buying at a store in-person, ask to be sized to ensure good fit. You can find nursing bras online at:

www.biggerbras.com
www.breakoutbras.com
www.decentexposures.com
www.ecobaby.com
www.growinglife.com

Goddess, Medela and Ameda brands offer large sizes. You can also have one custom-made by Jeunique International (*www.jeunique.com*).

Nursing clothes are available in plus-sizes at:
www.babybecoming.com
www.growinglife.com
www.mommygear.com
www.motherwear.com

When shopping for nursing clothes, look for slits that are large enough to accommodate your breasts without having to expose a lot of other skin. If there are buttons or snaps, make sure they are easy to operate one-handed. You might find that it's just easier to skip nursing clothes and lift up your shirt and use a blanket to cover yourself if you are in public. It can be a lot to manage to find the slit, get it open, reach through, get the bra flap open, move the pad out of the way, and pull the breast out through the slit with a screaming baby on your lap.

If you're interested in sewing your own nursing clothes, *www.eliza-bethlee.com* has plus-size patterns. You can also find out how to convert any shirt into a nursing shirt at *http://web.winco.net/~sbcortlu/makey-ourowntee.htm.*

If you have large breasts, you may need to purchase a breast pump that comes with a larger flange. Medela and Ameda brands now offer them. *Babybecoming.com* carries a larger-size nursing pillow.

For a detailed review of a variety of baby slings by a plus-size mom, see *www.thebabywearer.com/articles/WhatToO/PlusSizes.htm.* In general, when shopping for a sling or baby carrier, try it on before purchasing. Some are simply not made to accommodate a plus-size mom. Look for slings and carriers that are adjustable and padded.

"I bought some nursing nightgowns, but ended up not using them very often. My breasts were really leaky, and there was no way to go to bed without a bra and breast pads on. If I wore that under my nightgown, it was too hard to find the slit, get it open, and then reach in and unhook the bra and take out the pad."—Brenda M.

"I found nursing bras to be expensive, awkward, and uncomfortable. I wore my regular bras, but used a bra extender (the kind that costs seventy-nine cents at your local fabric store). That made it possible for me to pull it up when it was time for the baby to nurse."—Rita F.

"I did have trouble finding bras—42DD. The only place I could find nursing bras was Wal-Mart, and they fell apart after a month or so, but they were inexpensive, so I bought three at a time."—Vanessa R.

"I found that the popular Boppy [nursing] pillows would not fit around me, but that the Hugster—which has longer Velcro straps—worked perfectly."—Carla R.

"The biggest baby sling I found was still too small. So we returned it and didn't use it at all."—Julie M.

"I bought a couple of plus-size nursing shirts at Motherwear, but found they were too much of a pain compared to a regular shirt and light blanket."—Andrea H.

"J.C. Penney has the best bra section. No problems finding the right size."—Amelia M.

"I used to use nursing clothes, but got tired of them, especially if there were fasteners to undo. Since I usually wear T-shirts or sweatshirts anyway, it is just as easy to lift the shirt and use the loose fabric to cover my breast. I can't rave enough about my Maya Wrap! I got a large, and it is more than adequate. I have used various slings, and they fit OK, but would pull at my neck as the baby grew. The Maya wrap is still comfortable."—Margie P.

"I bought a nursing bra at a breastfeeding store where they supply all different products for breastfeeding. I was measured, and they actually had my size in stock."—Deb P.

Your Diet is Your Baby's Diet

OK, so once you get through pregnancy, your body is your own again, right? Well, if you're breastfeeding, it's not completely yours again while you're nursing. Your diet controls the nutrients your baby gets through your milk, so you should still be concerned about eating healthy. Talk with your health-care provider about what foods, medications, and supplements to avoid while nursing.

Nursing and Weight Loss

Breastfeeding can be a great way to lose weight, although some moms find it harder to lose weight while nursing than others. Lindsey-Salvo says that plus-size moms should eat 500 more calories a day while nursing and avoid strict weight-loss diets.

A study in the *New England Journal of Medicine* in 2000 concluded that it is safe for overweight moms to slowly lose weight while breast-feeding. According to the study, it is safe to cut down on fat and sugar intake (participants in the study cut their calories by 500 per day) when the baby is one month old. A weekly weight loss of one pound had no effect on babies between four and fourteen weeks old (the time period studied) and supplemental formula was not needed. The moms in the study reported having more energy because they exercised four times per week (they started by walking fifteen minutes a day and increased to forty-five minutes a day). The average weight loss was 10.5 pounds over the ten weeks of the study.

The key to successful breastfeeding is a happy and healthy mother. If you are stressed out over whether you managed to lose a pound this week, you aren't going to be as successful at nursing as you might otherwise be. You already know you should lose weight, but you might find that nursing is such a life change and such an energy drain that you just can't think about weight loss while you're doing it. Give yourself time, and don't pressure yourself. If you want to lose weight, you will when you're ready. Making yourself miserable about it now is just going to make you feel worse about yourself and make it harder for you to focus on nursing.

"I thought the nursing would take off all my extra sixty or seventy pounds, but alas, it didn't. After three months, I went on a diet. Happily, two years later, I've lost the extra weight."—Liz R.

"Everyone always said how nursing was a great way to lose weight. Ha! I felt like nursing really reduced my activity level because I was always sitting down to breast-feed and never had time to be active or do anything. I felt like a prisoner sometimes—always having to be near the baby to be able to feed. So, no, I didn't really lose a lot of weight while breastfeeding. It made me hungry, too. I don't know if it was just psychological, but I felt hungrier when breastfeeding than during pregnancy. If you think about it, your body is providing complete nourishment for the baby, which is even bigger and needs even more calories than it did while it was inside you."—Gail D.

Staying Comfortable

If you experience sore nipples, try Lansinoh cream, cold cabbage leaves, and air-drying your nipples after feedings. Nipple shields may work if you are having a serious ongoing problem, but many women find them uncomfortable. Your lactation consultant can be a great resource, so don't hesitate to ask if you're having problems. If you develop thrush, a yeast infection on the nipples (and usually in the baby's mouth as well), contact your pediatrician and your health-care provider.

If your nursing bra is cutting into your shoulders, back, or sides, take it off for a couple of hours, or buy several brands, and switch between them. Look for a bra with padded shoulder straps.

Leaky breasts are another problem with breastfeeding. Wear breast pads inside your bra, and change them at each feeding. Take extra pads with you if you go out. If you find your breasts are leaking, applying gentle pressure from the front and pressing toward your chest cavity can get it to stop. If your breasts leak during sex and that bothers you, wear a bra during intercourse, or keep breast pads close at hand so you can apply pressure if a leak develops.

If you have large breasts, you might develop skin problems on the bottom side of your breasts or where your breast and abdomen meet. This can be a problem particularly if you live in a warm climate or nurse in the summer. Moisture gets trapped under the breast and can cause rashes or topical yeast infections. Avoid using soap or other commercial products on your breasts, and instead, just wash with water and dry gently. Wash your bra frequently in hot water, and use bleach in the wash cycle to help kill any bacteria or remove milk stains. Allow air to circulate around your breasts, even if it means lying down and just holding them up. If you have a rash or irritation that won't go away, consult your health-care provider. He or she can prescribe topical treatments.

16

You Ain't Seen Nothin' Yet:
Life After Birth

After your baby is born, you'll be focused on your new role as mom to this wonderful little creature. Even though you'll be busy and happy, it's easy to spend too much time feeling bad about yourself and your weight. Your body created and gave birth to your amazing child. It was a long, long process and you can't expect to have a body resembling your prepregnancy one for a long time—and maybe never. The good news is that when you have the baby, you'll immediately lose a lot of weight. What a joy it is to step on the scale and see that you lost ten or 12 pounds! But, that joy can be clouded when you look at yourself in the mirror and wonder if you'll ever have a body you recognize again.

Your Postbirth Body

Once your baby is born, you'll feel much lighter, although you might miss that moving bump on the front of you. Your postpregnancy body is not going to look like your prepregnancy body, at least not for a while. Lots of women reported being unpleasantly surprised at what their postbirth bodies looked like. We see lots of photos of glowing pregnant women, but none of lumpy, saggy, hormonal, postnatal women. No one likes what they look like after just having had a baby, and the important thing to remember is that time will bring some changes, and your body will slowly adjust to having given birth.

Immediately after the birth, you'll be about the size you were in the middle of your pregnancy. The baby might be gone, but your uterus is still expanded and your abdomen is still enlarged. Probably the worst news is that your stomach is going to sag. You know how a balloon gets lumpy and floppy and loses its elasticity after you let the air out? The same thing will happen with your tummy. It's been stretched out holding your baby. Suddenly the baby's gone, but your tummy's still stretched out.

Your face might begin to look thinner as you lose some weight after the birth, and you'll find that your tummy will gradually shrink. Pregnancy stretches out your skin and muscles, so your tummy will probably never be as tight as it was before pregnancy. You might find that you have a flap of skin that hangs down in the front or that your weight has redistributed itself around your hips or to your stomach area. Stretch marks are inevitable for most women and will fade from red to a shade closer to your skin color in time. Creams that claim to reduce them have no effect.

Your breasts will get engorged when your milk comes in and will be simply huge and sore for a few days until the milk supply evens out. They'll stay large while you're nursing and then become smaller once you stop, although you can probably expect some sagging afterward. Many women report that after they stop breastfeeding, their breasts point straight down and seem to lose their perkiness.

These changes are all completely normal and other women (even thin women) experience them, as well. Be patient with your body, and give it time to recover from the very taxing experience of being pregnant and giving birth.

"So much sagging fat now. At least before it was tighter and could be hidden in clothes."—Peggy M.

"I felt like my belly was just dangling from my body all soft and mushy, but it sprang back up quite a bit. Do the exercises the doctor sends home with you, and you will do fine."—Jen R.

"It was actually more difficult for me *after* the pregnancy. I was the same weight as I was before, but now everything has shifted three inches south. I feel like I have all these rolls and really droopy breasts. I am still working on trying to feel good about my postbaby body. Hopefully your partner will tell you how attractive he still finds you, but I am my own worst critic. All I can say is that your body got this way because you created and nurtured new life, and if a few stretch marks and sags are the result of that miracle, so be it."—Carla R.

"I felt pretty badly about my body—now I was not only overweight, but my stomach hung lower than ever."—Dana C.

"When I saw some of those pictures of me, almost naked, giving baby a bath or whatever, I felt like I wanted to burn the negatives."—Amanda F.

"After my first baby was born and she was about seven months old someone asked me when I was due. I told them seven months ago and smiled. That shut them up."—Angie G.

"Recognize that you will never have the same body you once had. I weigh less now than I did prior to baby number one, but I cannot wear clothes from prebaby number one. The weight redistributes after a baby. Your hips may be slightly wider, for example. But then, having a baby changes you. It's only fitting that your body reflect that change."—Michelle C.

"I felt like I had a huge inner tube around me. My lower belly area was very heavy, and I was very aware of it. It felt different. I did feel bad about it."—Melissa S.

"My back does a big shift after birth, and often I have painful realignment for a few weeks. I worry a little bit about that. I also don't like looking four months pregnant when I'm not. I dislike the loose skin more than the weight."—Amelia M.

"I had always been overweight, but now I sagged on top of that! It's hard to see that sometimes, but mothers are always making sacrifices for their children, and I guess it starts with changes to our figure. One thing I regret was not wearing a bra all the time after the baby was born. When the milk came in and my breasts were huge, I should have had a really good support bra. Maybe that would have helped with some of the sagging later so I wouldn't be a thirty-three-year-old with the breasts of a sixty-three-year-old! But my kids bring so much joy to my life that it was worth whatever changes I went through. Besides, that's what Wonderbras are for."—Beth U.

Weight Loss

Some women are dying to lose weight after the baby, while others don't feel any great pressure. Whatever you want to do is OK. Don't feel pressured into insane dieting when you have so many new stresses. The key is to give yourself time to adjust to life as a mom before putting pressure on yourself to lose weight, if that's your goal. Some women find it impossible to lose weight while they are caring for an infant and find that they are more able to focus on themselves when the baby is older and more mobile.

If you want to lose weight, don't put yourself on a strict diet, particularly if you are breastfeeding. (See Chapter 15 for more information about weight loss and breastfeeding.) Dieting can reduce milk supply, and larger women are already at risk for low milk supply. Some women find they put on weight while breastfeeding and take it off once the baby is weaned. Don't panic if you're still breastfeeding and have weight you would like to lose. *Eat Well, Lose Weight While Breastfeeding* by Eileen Behan (Villard, 1992) is a book recommended by La Leche League.

Give yourself at least several months to initially recover from the birth and pregnancy. Your focus should be on your baby, not on the scale. Eating healthy will give you more energy and stamina and can help you lose weight. Any weight loss after birth should be slow and gradual. Sleeplessness, stress, and exhaustion can be big reasons for overeating. When you're exhausted, but you're up with the baby, or you finally got the baby to sleep, sometimes sitting down with a snack to relax would just feel so good. If you want to lose weight, try to eat on a schedule so you don't find yourself eating without thinking. The National Institutes of Health says that in general, a realistic weight loss goal is a 10-percent loss over a six-month period, so keep that in mind.

If you want to exercise, resume it gradually. Two to four weeks after a vaginal delivery and four to six weeks after a C-section are usually recommended, but talk to your health-care provider. If you notice an increase or resumption of vaginal bleeding during or right after exercise, you need to wait a few more days before trying again. Lisa Stone, ACE fitness expert and creator *of Fit for 2 Step Aerobic Workout for Pregnancy* (*www.fitfor2.com*), points out, "Remember, it takes nine months to put on the weight gained during pregnancy. It can take nine to twelve months after childbirth to lose that weight. Be patient!"

It can also be really hard to make time to exercise after having a baby when you can't even find time to take a shower. Walking can sometimes work well because you can do it with the baby. Although, it can be frustrating to take an invigorating walk during which the baby sleeps and then come home and want to rest, only to have a crying baby that needs attention. You might want to try an exercise video that you can start and stop as you need to throughout the day. If you have exercise equipment at home, this can also be a good way to gradually ease back into things. It's not advisable to use exercise equipment while wearing the baby in a sling.

A recent study from the University of Chicago and Stanford University has shown that lack of sleep increases hunger and appetite (increased desire for high-sugar, high-salt, and starchy foods) and results in weight gain. People who sleep less than eight hours a night are heavier than people who get enough sleep. New moms are definitely short on sleep, so you may find that you're hungrier than ever after your baby is born, and weight loss may feel impossible. Get as much sleep as you can. Remember that your baby is going to be small for a short time, and things will get better. You will, at some point, actually sleep through the night again! If you're sleep deprived, it's going to be very difficult to lose weight. Don't expect too much of yourself.

The key to weight loss and exercise after a baby is to have patience with yourself and to take small steps toward your goal. And if you feel like losing weight or implementing an exercise program isn't going to work for you at this point in your life, forgive yourself. Wait awhile, and try again later. If weight loss was something that was hard for you before the baby, you shouldn't expect it to be any easier after the baby—in fact, you should expect it to be even more difficult. Be realistic, and don't attempt to do more than you can handle because, ultimately, it will make you feel negative about yourself. Don't assume, however, that just because you can't take off the weight in the first six months that it is a lost cause. The important thing is that you have grown this incredibly gorgeous baby inside your body. Taking back your body will be a slow process, and you must have patience.

"I gained forty pounds after the baby was born. It was even more difficult to move around after the C-section."—Peggy M.

"I [went] back to my original weight, but I have been stuck there since then. I am trying to lose more."—Carla R.

"I did lose weight—about fifteen pounds, but then another ten or so over the next few months. I always seemed to reach my prepregnancy weight with relative ease; however, that weight was overweight."—Dana C.

"I dropped to my prepregnancy weight, but it all crept back on within two years of giving birth."—Sharon L.

"I did begin a weight-loss diet when my son was a couple months old and had fantastic success with it. Mainly, the thing was to keep it balanced and make sure I always ate the portions designed for lactating women."—Amanda F.

"I made the mistake of thinking that just running after my first son would slim me in a couple months. I only lost half the weight I gained."—Cheryl H.

"I didn't lose any weight after baby one. After baby two, I lost all that weight and half of the pregnancy before's weight within one year and six weeks. Baby number three, I lost the weight, but only after three years. Don't expect it to happen quickly. It took nine months to put it on, plan on at least a year from the time the doctor releases you to lose it. Watch your calorie intake very carefully. After eating for two, it's a hard transition."—Michelle C.

"I started to walk every day with my daughter in her Baby Bjorn. The pounds just started to melt off, and I was smaller than before I was pregnant in just four months."—Dana W.

"I missed the pregnancy status—back to being just fat. I gain very little during pregnancy, but usually gain after I deliver—careless eating and little sleep equals weight gain. Each time I vowed to be better, but it usually took a good nine to twelve months before I could focus on my own health."—Margie P.

"I lost two dress sizes after my first child. You just have to get out there and get active. Take your new baby for a stroll around the neighborhood every day. Park farther away from the entrance of buildings. Get a bike with a baby seat and a really cushy seat, and ride it to the park."—Ali S.

"I lost forty pounds relatively easily without working out or dieting, from nursing I believe, but now, eighteen months later, I am dieting and joining the gym. I am really down about it, but I just keep plugging away."—Vanessa R.

Your Future Weight and Health

If you gain more than the recommended amount of weight during pregnancy, or don't lose pregnancy weight in six months, studies have shown you are likely to carry at least an extra twenty pounds ten years after the birth. Keeping the weight on for more than six months also increases the amount of fat in your abdomen and ups your risks for diabetes and heart disease.

A University of Alabama at Birmingham study found that obese women were at greater risk for weight gain after pregnancy than thinner women. The study concluded that this was due to lifestyle changes, not physical reasons. Having a baby does change your life entirely. Part of the problem is that while you feel you are busier than ever, you may actually be less physically active. Rocking and pacing are movement, but they aren't the same as other exercise, and you're probably often too tired to do real exercise. Who can blame you? New motherhood takes a lot out of you. If you're having a terrible time losing weight after your baby is born, maybe it would be more useful to simply try to maintain your weight and worry about weight loss a little later, if it's something you want to achieve.

You know how much you weigh, you know that it's probably not the healthiest thing in the world, but you also know there are worse things. Beating yourself up about your body isn't going to make you feel any better, and you're not going to be a very happy mother if you spend the rest of your life obsessing over it. Do what you can to stay healthy and if losing weight is a goal, then go after it. Get professional help if you're serious about it and having trouble on your own. You're a grown-up and you understand perfectly well what an ideal body weight is, but you also know what is possible for you and what is not, at least right now.

Loving Your Postpartum Body

Perhaps the most-important thing to remember is that you're now a role model for your baby. Your baby is going to learn how to care for himself and think about himself based on how he sees you treat yourself. If you hate your body and are constantly talking about how awful it is and how disgusted you are with it, your child is going to learn to dislike his body, no matter how perfect it may be. The best thing you can do as a parent is to emphasize healthy habits and positive self-image. You may not be perfect, but at least you love and respect yourself for who you are.

"Just love your body. Because if you love your body, your kids will learn to love their bodies, and that's really the most important thing."—Liz O.

Co-Sleeping

The American Academy of Pediatrics (AAP) has changed its policy about co-sleeping, or sharing a bed with your baby. The AAP previously opposed it, even though in most countries throughout the world, parents and babies share beds on a regular basis. The AAP was concerned about risks to the baby, like being smothered or falling out of bed. The AAP has now carefully changed its policy to say, "Mother and infant should sleep in proximity to each other to facilitate breastfeeding."

If you read about co-sleeping in your parenting or baby care books, you'll see that the benefits of it are usually discussed, then situations in which you should not co-sleep are listed. This list will usually say that obese (sometimes this is limited to extremely obese parents) should not sleep with their babies. This is in addition to other situations, like smoking, taking drugs, or being under the influence of alcohol.

Co-sleeping is something that many parents feel very strongly about, and it's a good idea to discuss it with your pediatrician before making a decision. However, it's downright insulting to imply that simply because a mother is larger, she cannot sleep safely in the same bed as her baby—as if a woman who is larger than a size 5 might mistakenly crush her child in her sleep or not realize that her body is touching the baby. And it is insulting to imply that being overweight is in some way the same as using drugs or getting drunk.

The AAP has not gone so far as to actually endorse mom and baby sharing a bed, but the updated policy encourages parents to find ways to sleep near their baby, whether the baby is in a bassinet next to the bed or in a special crib (called a sidecar crib) that attaches to the side of the bed. A sidecar can give you the best of both worlds. Your baby is an arm's length away from you, and you can nurse and sleep at the same time. You don't have to feel crowded or worry about the baby falling over the edge.

Co-sleeping is an important way to make breastfeeding easier. Talk to your pediatrician, and make a decision that's right for you. If you choose to co-sleep, follow these tips:

- If you use a sidecar crib, make sure it is designed for this purpose and installed correctly
- If you choose to use your bed as a family bed, make sure the mattress is firmly against the headboard, and if one side is against a wall, make sure there is no space between it and the wall
- Avoid using heavy blankets
- Don't dress the baby in too many layers
- Keep pillows or comforters away from the baby
- Keep stuffed animals out of the bed
- Be absolutely certain that there is no way the baby can fall or roll off the edge of the bed

"With both kids, we had them in the bed with us in the beginning. It was so much easier to feed at night. I knew that doctors were against it, and I felt guilty about it, but there was no way I could get up four times in the night to go get the baby. I just stayed awake when the baby was feeding on the outside edge and then put her in the middle when I was going to sleep. We have a queen-size bed, and that worked pretty well. I think a king would make it even easier. You could keep the pillows away then. I didn't know this about bigger women not supposed to do it. I don't see how it matters if you're a size 2 or a size 20. If you're stupid enough to roll over on the baby, it's a bad thing no matter how big you are."—Kathleen J.

Health Implications for Your Child
Big Babies
Many doctors assume that because you're plus size, you will have a large baby. This isn't a given. If you have gestational diabetes, there is an

increased risk of delivering a larger baby. When the mother's blood sugar is high, it means the baby is getting an increased supply of glucose, causing increased growth. The mother's weight is also a factor in affecting the baby's weight, but is not always a determining factor. Genetics play a large part in it. If you and/or your partner were large babies, there's a good chance you will have a big baby—and if you weighed more than eight pounds at birth, your risk of having a large baby is doubled.

Your race is important, too—children of Asian mothers tend to be smaller. The baby's sex and birth order are also important. Boys tend to be bigger than girls, and each successive child tends to be bigger than the one before it. Additionally, if you had a big baby before, the odds are that you will have other big babies. Women who gain a lot of weight during pregnancy can expect to have larger babies. A baby that goes past its due date is also more likely to be large.

Shoulder Dystocia

Shoulder dystocia occurs when a baby, usually because it is large (the medical term for a large baby is macrosomic), becomes stuck in the birth canal during delivery. Shoulder dystocia can lead to fractured clavicle, nerve damage, bruising, and breathing problems for the baby. To prevent this, many doctors prefer to deliver larger babies by C-section. In nondiabetic women, most babies who have shoulder dystocia emerge completely fine—often the shoulder dystocia in these babies is not because the babies are too large and occurs because of positioning or broad shoulders. Infants of diabetic or gestational diabetic women have a higher incidence of shoulder dystocia because their babies tend to have what is called central obesity—they have a larger torso and chest. It's important to understand that in non-diabetic pregnancies, 50 percent of shoulder dystocias occur in normal sized babies and most large babies do not have shoulder dystocia.

Generally, obstetricians do not recommend a C-section based on how big the baby seems to be by fundal height or by ultrasound (since this estimate may have a 10- to 20-percent margin of error), unless the sonogram estimates a weight that is quite large (more than 5,000 grams or eleven pounds). C-sections may be offered or suggested to women with diabetes or gestational diabetes even if their baby is estimated to be smaller than this, since the risk of shoulder dystocia and complications for the baby are much higher in this group of women.

Low Blood Sugar

Large babies of large moms are prone to low blood sugar after delivery, whether or not the mother had gestational diabetes. If you tested negative, you may wonder why your baby is reacting as if you did have gestational diabetes. The reasons for this aren't clear, though it may be a related subtle carbohydrate intolerance, which is not detected by the usual standards for gestational diabetes but that has a similar effect on the baby. Feeding the baby in the delivery room can sometimes prevent sugar levels from dropping, and continuing to feed every two to three hours can help stave off problems. The good news is that larger babies can sometimes sleep better. They may be more difficult to wake up (which may be good because they'll sleep through anything, but can be disturbing if you have trouble waking your child up). If you have a large baby, be sure to talk to your pediatrician about what is normal and discuss any concerns you might have.

Impact of Large Birth Size

If your baby is large, you might find that he stands out in the nursery and seems more fully formed than the other babies. Some large babies have thicker hair, better neck control, and louder cries. You may find, though, that your layette (newborn clothes) is useless. Clothing designed for a five- or six-pound baby is not going to fit your eight-, nine-, or ten-pound baby. You'll have to move straight to clothes in size three months. Likewise, newborn-size diapers are not going to fit either.

If you do have a big baby, it doesn't necessarily mean she'll be larger for the rest of her life, although there is evidence that if your baby is large for her age at six months, she has an increased risk of obesity as an adult. (This is true for boys, as well.) Also, a pattern of rapid weight gain in the first four months is associated with a risk of being overweight at age seven. Some good news though—large birth-weight babies actually have a lower risk of developing diabetes later in life than low birth-weight babies. Studies have shown that in low birth-weight babies, poor prenatal nutrition permanently affects the body's ability to produce enough insulin to regulate blood sugar.

If your baby is large, you can probably expect that people will assume it's somehow your fault—that you ate too much during pregnancy, gained too much, or didn't eat healthy foods. Don't let other people make you feel bad. The size of your baby is something over which you have very little control, and genetics is the biggest influence. Parents who have big babies report loving their baby's increased responsiveness and the way they are completely filled out—they have yummy rolls of baby fat and big sweet cheeks to kiss. Big babies are remarkable and beautiful, and you should not allow anyone to make you feel bad about the gorgeous child you produced.

"My baby was nine pounds, ten ounces. Doctors said this was due to my size. But my mother, who never weighed more than 170 pounds at nine months of pregnancy with all five of her children, had nine-plus pound babies. I've been told by my Ob/Gyn that some women just have bigger babies, regardless of their size. I was made to feel this was related to my size, regardless of not getting gestational diabetes and also that my husband and his sister were both eleven-pound babies at birth. Doctors and nurses seemed to be turning a blind eye since it was easier to blame my weight. My baby is still bigger (weight and height). He is twenty-six pounds at ten months, but he is also thirty-one-inches tall."—Julie M.

"When my second child was born he was quite large (nine pounds, nine ounces) and had to be in NIC for hypoglycemia (low blood sugar), which was probably due to my having an elevated blood sugar (although it was never during the GD screenings). I was devastated to think that my horrible eating habits and/or weight had caused my innocent little baby to suffer so early in life. This feeling was expanded when I received my baby's health history that read, 'Baby's hypoglycemia is due to mother's obesity.' I was furious. His low blood sugar did not necessarily have anything to do with my weight—it was my elevated blood sugar, many thin women can have, too."—Dana C.

"The doctor told me I was having a big baby, but he was wrong. My daughter was only seven pounds, ten ounces when she was born. To me, that's not a big baby at all. I do not believe just because you're an overweight woman, you will have a bigger baby."—Jennifer W.

"No one has said anything, but I can see from people's stares that they relate my size to my daughter's (nine pounds, four ounces)."—Sharon L.

"He was more than nine pounds, but my previous baby was more than ten pounds. I didn't hear that it was related to my size, but mostly to genetics."—Liz R.

"My baby was seven pounds, seven ounces. I did have to have a second ultrasound because my doctor thought the baby was going to be big because of how big I was measuring."—Tammy M.

"My son was nine pounds. My daughter was nearly eleven pounds. When my son was born, the doctor thought there might have been some undiagnosed pregnancy diabetes, but this was never confirmed, and it wasn't repeated during my second pregnancy, although I was tested for it."—Amanda F.

"My third child was ten pounds, one ounce, and two weeks late. I felt like 'Oh geez, I'm so big, and I gave birth to a big baby!'"—Lisa B.

"Both my babies were on the larger side, eight pounds, fourteen ounces and nine pounds, nine ounces. I am pretty sure it was due to my size and eating habits. To me, bigger babies looked very healthy at birth, fuller looking. And after birth, they have grown very normally. They are even smaller than children smaller than them at birth."—Jennifer H

Your Baby's Health

Even if your baby is not large at birth, you might be wondering if your size has any kind of impact on him. A study from the University of Pennsylvania showed that children of overweight mothers are fifteen times more likely to be obese at age six. The study found that there were dramatic changes in body fat between ages three and six. Parents should be aware that this a key time to pay attention to your child's nutrition, weight, activity level, and health. This finding also indicated that much of this increase in body fat in the three-to-six-year range is due to genetics. The study did show that lower family income was tied to higher weight for the children. Children whose families had higher incomes tended to weigh less than children born into lower-income families.

You might read this information and feel helpless and guilty. The best way to look at it is that yes, if you're overweight, your child has a higher chance of being overweight, too. However, as the mom, you're probably the one in your family in charge of nutrition and a lot of parenting decisions, meaning that you have a lot of control. There's nothing you can do about a genetic predisposition in your family toward being overweight (just like there would be nothing you could do if your family had a genetic disposition for Alzheimer's or breast cancer). All kids are going to have higher risks of something. The good news is you now know about these risks and you can work to try to raise a healthy child. There's no reason to feel guilty or upset. No one in this world is perfect, and we take our lives and our bodies as they come to us. But, you can focus on being a parent who tries to manage these risks for your child. Have a conversation with your pediatrician about these risks and try to remain positive.

"I have more fears about my children growing up heavy like me than being heavy and pregnant. Also, I think a lot of people think or assume my children will be overweight growing up because I am, and sometimes this really makes me mad."—Jennifer H.

Life as a Plus-Size Mom

Life as a plus-size mom carries some additional challenges. There are so many things you will want to experience with your child and share with him or her. Being plus size shouldn't stop you from doing those things. Some moms worry about not being able to go on playground equipment with their kids or not being able to run fast enough behind a bicycle or about the looks they will get from other parents. First of all, public playground equipment is meant for kids, not adults, but even so, it's all made sturdily enough to hold an adult—even a large one. Don't let your size intimidate you. Go in the wading pool with your toddler, run around the playground, and simply be an active part of your child's life. What other people think doesn't matter—what does matter is being an active and involved parent. Your child doesn't know and won't care what size you are, but he or she will care if you hold yourself back and shy away from activities because of your size or self-image.

"I grew up with a mother who had been fat all her life. She was determined to make sure I was happy with who I was and how I looked. She never put me on a diet or made me feel bad, but was very encouraging when I did diet. This has set me up for a lifetime of being happy with myself. I am forever grateful for my mother for that gift, and I can only hope I can do the same for my daughter."—Tammy M.

"When my kids were little, I would never pose for any pictures with them because I hated the way I looked in the photos. After awhile, I realized that I had no photos of myself either with or without my kids. If something were to happen to me, they wouldn't even have a picture to remember me by! Now I refuse to be so self-conscious and will pose for a nice family picture every now and then. I even display a few of them."—Beth U.

"Don't ever let anyone tell you that size matters when you're a parent. You will experience the same highs and lows, joys and disappointments that thin parents experience and your size will impact little of your abilities as a parent. Sure, you may not be able to run the 100-meter dash in under ten seconds, but if you can make that journey in your own good time and with a smile, your kids will love you all the same. Big is beautiful—and that's the message we need to take to the world."—Sharon L.

Resource Appendix

Pregnancy books
Breastfeeding
The American Academy of Pediatrics New Mother's Guide to Breastfeeding by American Academy of Pediatrics (Bantam, 2002)

The Breastfeeding Answer Book by Nancy Mohrbacher (La Leche League International, 2003)

The Womanly Art of Breastfeeding: Seventh Revised Edition by La Leche League International (Plume, 2004)

C-sections
Cesarean Recovery by Chrissie Gallagher-Mundy (Firefly Books Ltd., 2004)

The Essential C-Section Guide: Pain Control, Healing at Home, Getting Your Body Back—and Everything Else You Need to Know About a Cesarean Birth by Maureen Connolly (Broadway Books, 2004)

What If I Have a C-Section? by Rita Rubin (Rodale Books, 2004)

Doulas

The Doula Advantage: Your Complete Guide to Having an Empowered and Positive Birth with the Help of a Professional Childbirth Assistant by Rachel Gurevich (Prima Lifestyles, 2003)

Exercise

Pilates for Pregnancy by Michael King (Ulysses Press, 2002)

General Pregnancy

A Child is Born by Lennart Nilsson (Delacorte Press, 2003)

The Mother of All Pregnancy Books by Ann Douglas (John Wiley & Sons, 2002)

The Pregnancy Bible by Joanne Stone (Firefly Books Ltd., 2003)

Pregnancy Sucks: What to Do When Your Miracle Makes You Miserable by Joanne Kimes (Adams Media Corporation, 2003)

The Thinking Woman's Guide to a Better Birth by Henci Goer (Perigee Trade, 1999)

Your Practical Pregnancy Planner: Everything You Need to Know About the Financial and Legal Aspects of Planning for Your New Baby by Brette McWhorter Sember (McGraw-Hill, 2005)

Your Pregnancy Week by Week, Fifth Edition by Dr. Glade B. Curtis and Judith Schuler, M.S. (Da Capo Press, 2004)

Nutrition

Eating for Pregnancy: An Essential Guide to Nutrition with Recipes for the Whole Family by Catherine Jones (Marlowe & Company, 2003)

Every Woman's Guide to Eating During Pregnancy by Martha Rose Shulman and Jane L. Davis, M.D. (Houghton Mifflin, 2002)

Nutrition for a Healthy Pregnancy, Revised Edition: The Complete Guide to Eating Before, During, and After Your Pregnancy by Elizabeth Somer, M.A., R.D. (Owl Books, 2002)

Postpregnancy

Outsmarting the Female Fat Cell After Pregnancy: Every Woman's Guide to Shaping Up, Slimming Down, and Staying Sane After the Baby by Debra Waterhouse (Hyperion Books, 2003)

This Isn't What I Expected: Overcoming Postpartum Depression by Karen R. Kleiman, M.S.W., and Valerie D. Raskin, M.D. (Bantam, 1994)

Sex

Hot Mamas: The Ultimate Guide to Staying Sexy Throughout Your Pregnancy and the Months Beyond by Lou Paget (Penguin USA, 2005)

Plus-size Books

The Big Girls' Guide to Life: A Plus-Sized Jaunt Through a Body-Obsessed World by Bunkie Lynn (Ladybug Llc, 2003)

Big Fat Lies: The Truth About Your Weight and Your Health by Glenn A. Gaesser (Gurze Books, 2002)

Bountiful Women: Large Women's Secrets for Living the Life They Desire by Bonnie Bernell (Wildcat Canyon Press, 2000)

The Fat Girl's Guide to Life by Wendy Shanker (Bloomsbury USA, 2004)

FAT!SO?: Because You Don't Have to Apologize for Your Size by Marilyn Wann (Ten Speed Press, 1999)

Just the Weigh You Are: How to Be Fit and Healthy, Whatever Your Size by Steven Jonas, M.D., and Linda Konner (Houghton Mifflin, 1998)

Learning Curves: Living Your Life in Full & with Style by Michele Weston (Crown, 2000)

Life is Not a Dress Size: Rita Farro's Guide to Attitude, Style, and a New You by Rita Farro (Chilton Book Company, 1996)

Nothing to Lose: A Guide to Sane Living in a Larger Body by Cheri K. Erdman (HarperSanFrancisco, 1996)

Real Fitness for Real Women: A Unique Workout Program for the Plus-Size Woman by Rochelle Rice (Warner Books, 2001)

True Beauty: Positive Attitudes and Practical Tips from the World's Leading Plus-Size Model by Emme (Perigee Books, 1998)

Wake Up, I'm Fat! by Camryn Manheim (Broadway, 2000)

Well Rounded: Eight Simple Steps for Changing Your Life . . . Not Your Size by Catherine Lippincott (Pocket Books, 1998)

What to Do When the Doctor Says It's PCOS: (Polycystic Ovarian Syndrome) by Milton Hammerly, M.D., and Cheryl Kimball (Fair Winds Press, 2003)

Web sites

Note to reader: If a direct link no longer works, go to the home page for the site, and search for the recommended topic or item.

Belly Casting
www.proudbody.com

Birth Defects
March of Dimes, *www.marchofdimes.com*
Birth Defect Research for Children, *www.birthdefects.org*
National Center on Birth Defects and Developmental Disabilities, *www.cdc.gov/ncbddd/*
National Birth Defects Prevention Network, *www.nbdpn.org*

Body Pillows
www.sitincomfort.com/comubodsuppi.html
www.mommysthinkin.com/serenity_star.htm
www.amazon.com/exec/obidos/tg/detail/-/B0000635WI/102-2870736-5916904?v=glance

Appendix

Breastfeeding
www.lalecheleague.org/llleaderweb/LV/LVMayJun89p35.html
     www.lalecheleague.org/llleaderweb/LV/LVAugSep00p63.html
http://health.groups.yahoo.com/group/MOBI/

Childbirth Education
International Childbirth Educators Association Inc., *www.icea.org*

Clothes (nonmaternity)
Catherine's Plus, *www.catherines.com*
Coldwater Creek, *www.coldwatercreek.com*
Draper' & Darnon's, *www.drapers.com*
Fashion Bug, *www.fashionbug.com*
Igigi, *www.igigi.com*
JMS: Just My Size, *www.justmysize.com*
Junonia, *www.junonia.com*
Lane Bryant, *www.lanebryant.com*
Making It Big, *www.makingitbigonline.com*
Plus Woman, *www.pluswoman.com*
Silhouettes, *www.Silhouettes.com*
Torrid, *www.torrid.com*
Ulla Popken, *www.ullapopken.com*
Zaftique, *www.zaftique.com*

Doppler for Home Use
www.bellybeats.com
www.healthchecksystems.com/babycom_doppler.htm
www.pregnancy-info.net/dopplers.html

Appendix

Doulas

DONA: Doulas of North American, *www.dona.org*

National Association of Postpartum Care Servers, *www.napcs.org*

Exercise During Pregnancy

Exercise tips, *www.babycenter.com/refcap/pregnancy/pregnancyfitness/
622.html*

In Fitness & In Health, *www.rochellerice.com*

The Big Mama Wellness Program, *http://thebigmama.com/*

Walking,
*http://health.discovery.com/centers/pregnancy/americanbaby/walk-
ing.html*

Stretching, *http://www.babycenter.com/refcap/588.html*

Fitness for pregnancy,
http://pregnancy.about.com/od/fitnesspregnancy/index_a.htm

Gestational Diabetes

American Diabetes Association, *www.diabetes.org/gestational-diabetes.jsp*

National Institute of Child Health & Human Development
Gestational Diabetes brochure,
www.nichd.nih.gov/publications/pubs/gest_diabetes.htm

About diabetes and pregnancy, *http://diabetes.about.com/od/gestational-
diabetes/*

High-Risk pregnancy

Sidelines National Support Network, *www.sidelines.org*

Jewelry for Pregnancy

Baby Chime Maternity Necklace, *http://pregnancy.about.com/cs/produc-
treviews/gr/aapr110603a.htm*

Charms and pendants, *www.beforebaby.com/index.php*
Pregnancy jewelry, *www.twinklelittlestar.com/us/pregnancy-jewelry.html*
Pregnancy jewelry, *www.attachmentscatalog.com/gifts/jsilver.html*

Maternity Clothes
BB Maternity, *www.bbmaternity.com*
Baby Becoming Maternity, *www.babybecoming.com*
Due Maternity, *www.duematernity.com*
Ebay, *www.ebay.com*
Fashion Bug, *www.fashionbug.com*
J.C. Penney, *www.jcpenney.com*
Jake and Me, *www.jakeandme.com*
Kmart, *www.kmart.com*
Maternity 4 Less, *www.maternity4less.com*
Maternity Clothing Fashions, *www.maternity-clothing-fashions.com*
Maternity Mall, *www.maternitymall.com*
Mom's Maternity, *www.momsmaternity.com*
Motherhood Maternity, *www.motherhood.com*
OPSS, OMOM's and Big Mom's Trading arena,
      www.network54.com/Forum/goto?forumid=14843
Pickles & Ice Cream, *www.plusmaternity.com*
Plus Mom Maternity, *www.plusmommaternity.com*
QVC, *www.qvc.com*
Sears, *www.sears.com*
Target, *www.target.com*
Wal-Mart, *www.walmart.com*

Undergarments
www.biggerbras.com
www.justmysize.com
www.pluswoman.com
www.growinglife.com

Waistband extensions
Bella Band, *www.bellaband.com*
*http://store.babycenter.com/product/clothing/moms_essentials/materni-
ty/5176 http://www.kidsurplus.com/maternity.html*

Midwives
The American College of Nurse-Midwives
www.acnm.org
240-485-1800

Midwives Alliance of North America
www.mana.org
888-923-MANA (6262)

North American Registry of Midwives
www.narm.org
888-842-4784

Nursing Bras, Clothes, and Equipment
www.babybecoming.com
www.biggerbras.com
www.breakoutbras.com
www.decentexposures.com
www.ecobaby.com
www.growinglife.com
www.jeunique.com
www.mommygear.com
www.motherwear.com

Appendix

Obstetricians
American College of Obstetricians and Gynecologists, *www.acog.org*

Plus-size Pregnancy
 http://pregnancy.about.com/od/plussizepregnanc/
www.plus-size-pregnancy.org
www.yourplussizepregnancy.com (the companion site to this book)

Plus-size Yellow Pages
www.plussizeyellowpages.com

Polycystic Ovarian Syndrome (PCOS)
www.4woman.gov/faq/pcos.htm
Polycystic Ovarian Syndrome Association (PCOSA), *www.pcosupport.org*
Hormone Foundation, *www.hormone.org*
Soul Cysters, *www.soulcysters.com*

Preeclampsia
Preeclampsia Foundation, *www.preeclampsia.org*

Preggie Pops
www.threelollies.com

Pregnancy Loss
www.pregnancyloss.info
National Stillbirth Society, *www.stillnomore.org*

Pregnancy Software
Baby Progress, *www.babiesonline.com/babyprogress*
Babystep, *www.babystep.com*
MomToBe, *www.storks-store.com/MomToBe/index.html*
Pregnancy Calendar, *www.tucows.com/preview/303153.html*

Relaxation Techniques
www.lhj.com/home/Relaxation-Techniques.html
http://stress.about.com/od/relaxation/

Scarf Tying
www.apparelsearch.com/scarve_knots.htm
www.dressingsmart.com/cart/index.php/item/department/ebooks/item/4.html

Sewing Patterns
http://patternsthatfityou.com/Maternity.htm
www.simplicity.com
www.isewplus.com
www.elizabethlee.com
http://web.winco.net/~sbcortlu/makeyourowntee.htm

Slings and Carriers
www.babybecoming.com
www.babysling.com
www.thebabywearer.com/articles/WhatToO/PlusSizes.htm
www.kangarookorner.com
www.mayawrap.com

Specialty Maternity Clothes (gowns, scrubs, suits, petite, tall)
www.babybecoming.com
www.jakeandme.com
www.jcpenney.com
www.maternity-clothing-fashions.com
www.plusmaternity.com
www.sassyscrubs.com
www.scrubs-r-us.com

Support and Listservs

BabyCenter plus-size pregnancy bulletin board,
    www.babycenter.com/bbs/8404/index.html

PCOS support, *www.soulcysters.net* and *www.pcossupport.org*

Plus-Size Pregnancy List Serv, *big_moms_list-request@lists.carrotpatch.net*
    Send an e-mail to the above address with a message of **subscribe
    big_moms_list**.

Trying to Conceive, Infertility, Pregnancy & Parenting Support for
    BBWs, *www.fertilityplus.org/bbw/*

Your Plus-Size Pregnancy, *www.yourplussizepregnancy.com*

Weight Issues

The American Obesity Association, *www.obesity.org*

International Size Acceptance Association, *www.size-acceptance.org*

National Association to Advance Fat Acceptance, *www.naafa.org*

Index

Index

Index

Index

Index

breasts, 226
C-section care, 203-204
   exercise, 229
   weight loss, 228-230
Preeclampsia, 38, 91-92
   and aspirin, 92
   and preterm birth, 93
   and vitamins, 91
   and weight gain, 57, 64
Preggie Pops, 16
Pregnancy induced hypertension, *see* hypertension
Pregnancy journal, 160
Prenatal classes, 167-171
   and birth ball, 170-171
   Bradley, 168
   combination, 168
   hypnobirthing, 168
   Lamaze, 168
   and nutrition, 171
   positions, 169
   refresher, 168
   VBAC, 168
   with spouse or partner, 165, 169
Pressure dressings, 202
Preterm
   birth, 93
   labor, 89
Progesterone, 209
Prolactin, 208, 209
Prolonged ruptured membranes, 189, 202
Progress, tracking, 158
Protein in urine, 91
Pulmonary embolism, 200
Pulse oximetry, 180
Pushing, 173

Quad screen test, 54, 101, 103

Reglan, 216
Relationships, nurturing, 115
Relaxing, 158-159
Respect, 138-139
Rewards, 137
Risk, 82-84
   coping with, 102-103

Salt, 19
Sequential or intermittent pneumatic compres-

sion devices, 201
Self-Esteem, 135-138, 232, 240
Self-image, *see* Self-Esteem
Scale in doctor's office, 36, 46
Screening tests, 47, 52-55
Scrubs, 132
Sea Bands, 16
Seatbelt extension, 20
Sewing, 129-130
Sex, 25-26
Shape change, 24-25
Shoes, 132-133
Shoulder dystocia, 95, 235-236
   and large-for-gestational-age babies, 236
Sibutramine, 103
Sidecar crib, 233-234
Size
   of baby, 38, *see also*, Large-for-gestational-age baby
   during pregnancy, 6
   separating from self, 6-8
Sleep, 23-24
   apnea, 94-95
   and nausea, 16
   and postpartum weight loss, 229-230
   with baby, 233-234
Sleepwear, *see* Clothing
Spandex, 119
Spina bifida, 52, 100
   Association, 100
   and ultrasounds, 50, 102
Spinal anesthesia
   and C-sections, 195-198
   comparison with epidural, 197
   and needle length, 181
Spirit, nurturing, 114-115
Spouse
   involving, 163-165
   and support, 146-148
Stillbirth, 38, 89, 96
Stretch marks, 226
Stretching, 21
Stress, 143
Success, 137
Suits, 132
Support, 145-154
Surroundings, 111
Syndrome O, *see* Polycystic Ovarian Syndrome

Index

About the Authors

Brette McWhorter Sember

Brette McWhorter Sember is a plus-size mom of two who felt it was time someone noticed the fact that half the pregnant women in this country are plus size! Sember is a former attorney and author of twenty nonfiction books, including *Your Practical Pregnancy Planner: Everything You Need to Know About the Financial and Legal Aspects of Planning for Your New Baby* (McGraw-Hill, 2005), *How to Parent With Your Ex: Working Together in Your Child's Best Interest* (Sourcebooks, 2005), and *The Complete Adoption and Fertility Legal Guide* (Sourcebooks, 2004). She has also written a children's book. Sember is a contributing writer for *ePregnancy* print magazine, a contributing editor to *amaZe* magazine and has written extensively about family and parenting. Her freelance work has appeared in more than 140 publications, including *Pregnancy, American Baby, Every Baby, Child,* and others. She is a member of the Association of Health Care Journalists (AHCJ) and the American Society of Journalists and Authors (ASJA). Her Web sites are *www.BretteSember.com* and *www.YourPlusSizePregnancy.com.*

Bruce D. Rodgers, M.D.

Bruce D. Rodgers, M.D., is a maternal-fetal medicine specialist with twenty years of clinical experience in the care of high-risk pregnancies. He is board certified in obstetrics and gynecology, and maternal-fetal medicine, and is a fellow of the American College of Obstetricians and Gynecologists. He is an associate professor of clinical obstetrics and gynecology at the State University of New York at Buffalo, School of Medicine and Biomedical Sciences, and is presently director of the Division of Maternal-Fetal Medicine and Fetal Cardiovascular Medicine at the Children's Hospital of Buffalo, in Buffalo, New York.